'I went (to Liz) for Craniosacral Therapy after suffering from a bad fall that had aggravated lumbar arthritis and after the failure of painful conventional treatments which hadn't provided any long-term relief. At first I was a little sceptical about the treatment but I found it to be relaxing, restoring and healing, and it has improved the quality of my life considerably. Reading this book reminded me of my own very positive experience of this work. No question, should the need arise, I shall return for more treatment.'

*– Chris McVie, Fleetwood Mac*

'Liz and Daška have presented a powerful journey through the personal and interpersonal processes that emerge as craniosacral sessions unfold and deepen. They stress that they are writing from a feminine perspective and that is so essential to hear and receive. Craniosacral work is essentially feminine in nature, based on states of presence, relationship and a deepening into a depth of listening and stillness. It is from this depth of presence, relationship and stillness, as the founder of the work, William Garner Sutherland, stressed, a deeper intelligence emerges and session work unfolds uniquely in each moment of time. I really appreciated the personal journeys described in this volume and hope it supports all readers in their own journey in life within the whole spectrum of joy, sorrow and healing processes.'

*– Franklyn Sills, Co-Founder and Co-Director of the Karuna Institute, author of* Foundations in Craniosacral Biodynamics

**EVERY
BODY
TELLS
A
STORY**

*of related interest*

**Getting Better at Getting People Better**
**Creating Successful Therapeutic Relationships**
*Noah Karrasch*
ISBN 978 1 84819 239 3
eISBN 978 0 85701 186 2

**The Compassionate Practitioner**
**How to Create a Successful and Rewarding Practice**
*Jane Wood*
ISBN 978 1 84819 222 5
eISBN 978 0 85701 170 1

**Cranial Intelligence**
**A Practical Guide to Biodynamic Craniosacral Therapy**
*Ged Sumner and Steve Haines*
ISBN 978 1 84819 028 3
eISBN 978 0 85701 012 4

# EVERY BODY TELLS A STORY

## A CRANIOSACRAL JOURNEY

Liz Kalinowska and Daška Hatton

Illustrated by Larry Vigon

SINGING
DRAGON
LONDON AND PHILADELPHIA

First published in 2016
by Singing Dragon
an imprint of Jessica Kingsley Publishers
73 Collier Street
London N1 9BE, UK
and
400 Market Street, Suite 400
Philadelphia, PA 19106, USA

*www.singingdragon.com*

**Library of Congress Cataloging in Publication Data**
Names: Kalinowska, Liz. | Hatton, Daška.
Title: Every body tells a story : a craniosacral journey / Liz Kalinowska and
    Daška Hatton.
Description: London ; Philadelphia : Singing Dragon, 2016.
Identifiers: LCCN 2015048219 | ISBN 9781848192683 (alk. paper)
Subjects: LCSH: Craniosacral therapy. | Therapeutics, Physiological.
Classification: LCC RZ399.C73 K35 2016 | DDC 615.8/2--dc23
LC record available at http://lccn.loc.gov/2015048219

**British Library Cataloguing in Publication Data**
A CIP catalogue record for this book is available from the British Library

ISBN 978 1 84819 268 3
eISBN 978 1 78450 281 2

Printed and bound in Great Britain

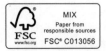

To our families and friends

# ACKNOWLEDGEMENTS

The authors would like to thank Larry Vigon for his art direction and design and Tom Hatton for his graphic design. All identifying characteristics and other details have been changed. We would like to thank those friends and colleagues who read our manuscript and gave such very helpful feedback.

# CONTENTS

# IN THE BEGINNING

We come to know ourselves through our sensory perceptions of life, how the world affects us and how we move within it. Our bodies are a map of our histories, the narrative of our lives; they record the ways in which we were brought up, they chronicle our accidents and illnesses, our emotional experiences and our beliefs. They reflect the stories we tell ourselves, and the stories others tell about us.

A course of treatment from a bodywork therapist can affect us in unexpected ways. What starts as a visit for a sore shoulder or a tendency to have headaches could become a journey into the heart of our emotional life and perhaps the depths of early experience. While the so-called mind/body connection is a familiar concept amongst therapists, it is not necessarily so obvious to the general public. One of our aims in writing this book is to highlight this vital connection and to show how it might manifest within the therapeutic context. Following the journey of a fictional client and therapist we show a relationship evolving and developing in 'real time': how the participants in the situation transform and grow through their interaction and how each of them contributes to the process. We have included our own experience of writing this book because, as it took shape, we found that it became yet another meaningful thread in our story.

The idea for this book grew slowly out of a friendship and an ongoing discussion of our work as Craniosacral Therapists and we decided we would like to give an account of the process that may be experienced during a course of therapeutic bodywork. As Craniosacral Therapists we have naturally used this discipline as the basis of the book, but we strongly believe that what follows will be equally relevant to other bodywork practitioners and their clients, as well as anyone interested in finding out more about the scope of bodywork.

Our intention is to demonstrate the mysterious and enchanting quality of Craniosacral Therapy, an experience unlike any other but not one that can be easily described in words. If asked for our explanation we would answer that most of our work is incredibly simple; we listen and offer rest and resourcing. It can often be mundane. We don't offer to cure or heal or see into the future or the past, but we do put our hands on people, and something happens when we do. Essentially, Craniosacral Therapy is a form of holistic bodywork, which has evolved from the teachings of both early and modern-day Osteopaths. As a structural model it is concerned with the central nervous system that runs between the cranium and the sacrum, its surrounding membranes and cerebrospinal fluids. However, even experienced practitioners find it hard to say exactly why or how it works. In textbooks you will find theories about fluid tides, body rhythms and fascial restrictions, all of which are influenced by the use of a light listening touch, magically restoring health. There is little actual evidence that this is the case. Our own conclusion, after many years of working in this field, is that a listening touch from an experienced practitioner can in fact alter things in the body, but primarily because it awakens a self-listening and healing in the client that does not necessarily or exclusively rely on any form of manipulation, however imperceptible.

In our opinion, connecting successfully with a client is the vital key to facilitating change. We believe that change is achieved through the development of a trusting relationship between client and practitioner, and the practitioner's skilful ability to reflect to the client where she may be holding tension or where there are restrictions in the body, either physical or emotional. It is very much a counselling of the body, bringing about relief by encouraging self-awareness and recognition of the source of a problem, and ultimately relying upon a growing appreciation by the client of her own powerful ability to heal.

From having been clients ourselves and working with colleagues, we know that practitioner and client can sometimes have completely different experiences during a treatment. We have learned that this in no way invalidates the process, but it does mean that we are often working totally in the dark. We may not know exactly why someone has come to see us and very often she doesn't either. While there might be an ostensible reason for the visit – a stiff neck, a frozen shoulder, a bad back – very often there is only a general feeling that things are not quite right and that our clients don't know which way to turn. We are frequently unsure how to work, what to say, where to put our hands. Sometimes we don't know if we have made a connection at all. Images, words, colours, snatches of song or music may come to us. Occasionally there is just silence. But now and then there is a glimpse of something greater than the two of us, and the world stops. Moments like this are indefinable and our story describes how such an experience might unfold.

When we first sat down together to put words on paper, it was because we saw that there was also a real need to give a woman's side of the story. A large percentage of practitioners and clients are women but their voices are not being heard clearly enough. Craniosacral Therapy is gentle and delicate by nature, and to celebrate these qualities, we thought that we would bring a female perspective to the table and share our journeys of discovery. It has been a long and interesting project, and our experience of writing has paralleled the voyage of discovery that you might undertake during a series of treatments. We have found it enjoyable, inspirational and frequently frustrating.

Although our focus throughout is on a feminine way of healing and how it might differ from the masculine, we are not arguing for an exclusively female perspective at the expense of the male. This is rather a plea to see the whole picture, to offer the possibility of reconnecting not only the masculine and the feminine but also the mind and the body. In this text we have tended to use the female pronoun as a corrective balance.

How then does the feminine perspective shape our work and in what way is this different from the masculine? In our view, the range of perception that belongs to female experience gives it a different dimension to the established masculine approach. Feminine energy is spacious, non-verbal, non-specific, relational and alchemical in nature. This is the archetypal female consciousness that has been celebrated throughout the ages. As women we are naturally attuned to the hidden energies and rhythms of life; as therapists we receive through our eyes and hands the ebbs and flows of inner tensions and listen to the inherent stories beneath the surface. The cycles of nature are consciously experienced by every woman from puberty; the knowledge that the flesh, and we ourselves, are subject to forces entirely beyond our control. We may have learnt how to control our hormones artificially, but essentially we are all subject to natural laws that remain beyond our present understanding. This understanding is fundamental to the feminine sensibility: we know in our bones, in our very essence, that 'man is not the measure of all things' and inevitably this is what we bring to the treatment room. As Craniosacral Therapists, both male and female, we offer a receptivity coupled with observation, an ability to wait without trying to influence the outcome. The conscious act of waiting for nature to take its course is intrinsic to the feminine; it is not based on passivity but on an active willingness to receive and brings us into contact with the mysterious, the numinous and the magical. We want to emphasise that this way of working is not unique to women and the searchlight of masculine intellect is of course just as essential to providing balance as the woman's diffuse and compassionate awareness. We could describe this masculine focus as concentration, but this implies a narrowing of perception to one point alone, whereas what we are looking for is exactly the opposite: a widening of concentration, an active attention.

We are not only seeking to cure symptoms, although this happens too, but to rebalance, to reconcile the opposites and to allow mutually exclusive truths to exist at the same time. The feminine approach to healing is to ask the restorative and compassionate question 'What ails thee?' and, more importantly, to listen to the answer. Listening at this deeper level can be the key to awakening a client's own experience of herself and her unacknowledged needs. We watch and wait for whatever may emerge.

We use the word 'healing' in this book in a very general sense and not to indicate any particular technique or procedure. Healing occurs in all the caring professions – conventional and alternative, medical or psychotherapeutic. So, what *do* we mean by healing? The World Health Organization defines health as 'a state of complete physical, mental, and social well-being and not merely the absence of disease or infirmity'[1]. The word healing literally means to 'make whole' or 'holy'. We ourselves make a distinction between healing and curing because we believe they are two very different things. We would argue that healing is the feminine way – an open and receptive

---

1    World Health Organization (1946) Preamble to the Constitution of the World Health Organization as adopted by the International Health Conference, New York, 19-22 June 1946, and entered into force on 7 April 1948.

approach that has no agenda. When we work with someone to bring about healing, we are working on a level that transcends superficial symptoms and aims to give power and responsibility to the receiver. Curing suggests to us a more masculine, proactive, approach that implies having something done to you; it takes responsibility away from the client and gives it to the practitioner. Little is learnt and a quick result is expected or promised, and this may be impossible to fulfil. In some cases the need to produce a cure may even obscure true healing and become the source of more disease. Our interest is primarily in a shared journey in which both practitioner and client are equally engaged, rather than in the traditional medical model. However, we do realise that our way of working is not always appropriate for everyone, and often traditional medical intervention is necessary.

The healing process we describe arises of its own volition out of the relationship between client and practitioner. As Craniosacral Therapists, we don't offer our clients a quick fix or an instant cure, but more importantly a chance to gain a greater understanding of themselves from a different perspective; an opportunity to see where they have come from and where they might go from here. Often, all that is required is a belief on the part of both that change may emerge from their particular connection. Healing is not to be rushed or hurried and relief of physical symptoms is not necessarily the only outcome; coming to terms with, and accepting responsibility for, our health and ourselves is as important. Good health, as defined earlier, is more than just the absence of symptoms.

This book is neither an attempt to validate bodywork using a scientific model nor a defence of the placebo effect. We are not suggesting that complementary medicine is the only way; since we are not scientists we do not aim to challenge the work of those who are. We believe that a course of therapeutic bodywork such as Massage, Rolfing, Craniosacral Therapy or the Alexander Technique can be as valuable and useful as undergoing a course of psychotherapy or conventional medicine, it all depends on 'What ails thee'. In our experience, therapeutic bodywork is extremely compatible with any of the talking therapies. In fact, it's possible that not to include the body might leave the analysand stuck in her head. Our aim as therapists is for any fundamental change in outlook or perspective to be grounded and embodied as opposed to remaining an intellectual construct on one level alone.

Rather than writing a manual of techniques and protocols, we wanted to present a more lyrical attempt to discover and illustrate the process of our work. Books about bodywork will often rely on perfunctory case histories to illustrate the process of the therapy, giving the impression that bodywork is a quick and easy solution to any number of ailments. This has not been our experience. We have found that change, where it occurs, is usually slower and very much less dramatic.

In our society we always seem to be searching for the ultimate healing answer. There are wounds that exist on the different planes of our mental, emotional, spiritual and physical lives and we suffer because of a disconnection between these different levels. In our work we are trying to find a balance between these various layers and by doing so to enlarge our perceptions of ourselves as part of something greater than our own stories. What we offer is a pathway that allows us to inquire more deeply, to look beyond the surface of our lives. It is exciting to discover the infinite possibilities of change. We like to imagine that our structures are fixed and that there are universal truths. We prefer to think that we have inherited our bad backs and our genetic constitutions and that we can't alter our environments. This is not necessarily so and the sense of freedom that this implies is dizzying. However old we are, we have the potential to change, grow and learn.

Another of our goals is to show how bodywork therapy actually works in the real world. After the training course is finished and a certificate awarded, the newly qualified bodywork therapist finds that practice essentially consists of two people alone in a room with one person touching the other. It is a relationship unlike any other and can be an astonishingly intimate connection. In any therapy the rapport between the two participants is central to the success or otherwise of the treatment, but none of the books that we have discovered so far tell the story as it develops on both sides of the table or describe what it is like to have a series of treatments from a Craniosacral Therapist. We hope that we show the alchemical transformation that can take place between the two participants, an element that is largely missing from other literature. We want to reflect the mysterious and inspirational quality of the work without losing sight of the everyday experience of being in practice.

We spent some time wondering how to bring all these different strands together in book form. At first we struggled with a format. The scholarly approach has already been well covered, and we don't feel we have anything further to contribute. We needed a different container for our own experience of Craniosacral Therapy and how it might develop over time. In order to do this we created two imaginary characters, Anna and Sarah, who would tell their own story. Our characters are not entirely fictional; between us we have been in practice for more than 40 years. In that time we have seen many Annas and often felt like Sarah. Anna, though, is not based on any one client; she is a fictitious woman who has come along for treatment with a familiar set of symptoms and case history. There is always a client like Anna, vulnerable and with a story so close to your own that it is hard to separate yourself from her. Sarah is neither one of us, nor even a combination of us both, but an invented therapist who encounters difficulties very much like those we have met over the years. Both characters have elements of each of us creeping in here and there, but that was inevitable. We have become quite fond of Anna and Sarah as we have gone along. The therapeutic process that we describe has, of necessity, been considerably telescoped and outcomes like these would almost certainly take much longer than ten sessions. In reality, a path like Anna's may need to be travelled for many months or even years.

Whilst writing we asked ourselves whether our characters, Anna and Sarah, rang true. How much of our own stories could we share? We eventually settled on a plan that would give both women a voice and allow us to explore, in fictional terms, the impact that each had on the other. Our framework also gave us the best opportunity to comment on the approach that our imagined therapist had taken and to show her struggles with her own process behind the scenes. In the beginning, however, it was hard for us to let our own voices come through clearly. We needed to find a way to bring our own experience into the picture. At first we tried to illustrate this by introducing a third fictional voice. Because our therapist sometimes talks about taking things to her supervisor we wanted to emphasise her role behind the scenes. This voice was quite capricious; it kept changing its personality and didn't really know who it was. Sometimes it sounded patronising and overbearing; at other times it was light and frivolous. Because it was so amorphous, we found the character much harder to name than we did Anna and Sarah. We didn't seem to be able to get in touch with her at all. At last we came to the decision that the third voice should be a combination of our own, as there was no reason for us to hide behind a fictional persona and we decided to act as observers in our commentary pieces.

We set out to show the impact of the relationship between the therapist and her supervisor on the progress of the treatment. Even though the client and supervisor never meet, she plays a large part in the dynamic of the treatment process. As in counselling and psychotherapy, a supervisor's role is to provide a space in which the practitioner can review and reflect on any aspect of her work. We want to use our story not only to demonstrate how valuable this tripartite relationship is to the treatment process but also to show that, like any other, it has its ups and downs. An awareness of the concepts of transference and counter transference is even more important for bodywork practitioners than it is for traditional talk-based psychotherapists, as the additional stimulus of touch and the felt sense adds more potential difficulties to negotiate. This different dimension brings its own characteristics and problems for a practitioner that need to be acknowledged. A supervisor offers feedback on anything that might arise and helps a practitioner to distinguish where she is falling into unhelpful patterns, crossing client/practitioner boundaries or getting too deeply involved. The supervisor is the third person in the treatment process, unseen by the client, but providing the balancing leg of the tripod.

We knew from the outset that we wanted to weave myths and archetypes into the book. Myths illustrating rites of passage occur in almost every culture; they are timeless and universal and represent a map for life. They aren't linear or logical progressions and they are discovered afresh and reinterpreted by each generation. They represent stages along the way where earlier travellers have left warnings of danger as well as encouragement to those who follow in their footsteps. A strong connection exists between these ancient narratives and our current emotional challenges. They are as relevant today as ever, perhaps even more so, since our culture is so rooted in a tendency towards abstract, rational and intellectual thought at the expense of the intuitive, symbolic or even mythic dimensions. We note that Jung wrote in the Commentary on the Secret of the Golden Flower in 1929, that 'the gods have become diseases; Zeus no longer rules Olympus but rather the solar plexus and produces curious specimens for the doctor's consulting rooms'.[2] This perfectly unites our interests and we felt that myths were an ideal way of explaining the underlying motives and behaviour of our protagonists.

We have based our story loosely on the stages of the Hero's Journey with its advances and setbacks, gains and losses. There are also echoes of Christian's adventure in John Bunyan's *The Pilgrim's Progress,* and of many other mythical odysseys. Two myths in particular seemed relevant. First, and most obvious, is the archetype of the Wounded Healer, which portrays the vulnerability of the therapist and its effects on both parties. Second, we have used the cyclical journey of growth and rebirth that is at the heart of the myth of Demeter and Persephone as an allegory of Anna and Sarah's relationship over the course of the treatments.

Nearly two years after we had begun, the book had taken its final shape.

---

2   Jung, C.G. (1938) Commentary on 'The Secret of the Golden Flower', Volume 13, *The Collected Works of C.G. Jung.* Princeton, NJ: Princeton University Press.

# CHAPTER ONE

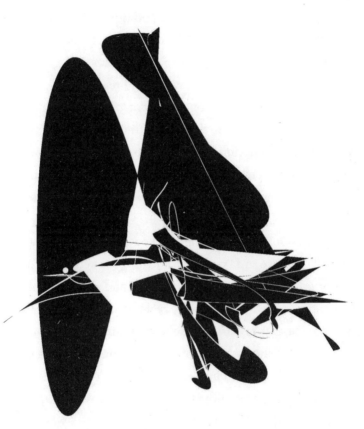

# DEPARTURE

## Anna's Story

I was feeling pretty nervous this morning as I approached Sarah's house for the first time. This was partly because I was running late as usual. The children were more difficult than ever this morning, and by the time I had got them off to school, there had been hardly any time left for me to shower, dress and tidy up the house before I was due to leave for my appointment. The traffic was really bad, and although I quickly found a parking space, I was still a few minutes behind time and very out of breath when I reached the door.

There was no number on the front of the building and no obvious clue to guide me to Sarah's treatment room, so I lost several more minutes wondering if I was in the right place and whether I should try the basement or the house upstairs. By this time, I was quite panicked and not sure whether to stay or just turn around and go home.

Finally I spotted a small sign tacked onto the wall outside the basement entrance and I ran down and rang the bell. Sarah answered the door immediately, introduced herself and showed me in to her treatment room. I didn't have any real preconceptions of what she would be like, but my first vague impressions were of a calm and friendly person who luckily didn't seem too put out by the fact I was late. She invited me to sit in a big comfortable chair by the window and I quickly shrugged off my coat, threw it over the arm and sat down, not wanting to waste any more of her time. I was cross with myself for being late, and still shaky and breathless, but although I desperately wanted to sit still and pay attention, I somehow found myself fumbling about in my handbag, switching off my phone, finding a tissue and finally managing to drop everything on the floor while Sarah patiently waited for me to settle down. Picking it all up took ages and made me so much more anxious and trembly that I found it extremely hard to finally sit back in the chair.

I didn't really know what to expect from the consultation, which was another reason I was so agitated. I had made the appointment about ten days ago as a result of talking to my friend, Sasha. I had been complaining to her recently about how tired, low in energy and stressed I was feeling. I was generally run down, and hadn't been properly well for some time. My symptoms kept changing. One day it was one thing, and the next it was something else. Nothing seemed to make any sense any more. Some days I felt so exhausted I just didn't want to get out of bed. On top of that, I was anxious about everything, even stupid little things that didn't matter. I honestly didn't know what was wrong with me. I had tried talking to my husband, Nigel, about it, but he'd just said perhaps I needed some vitamins or a day out somewhere, which wasn't much help. I was getting pretty desperate to feel better, and no one seemed to be listening to me. I had been to a doctor in the past and he had just told me that I was stressed and needed to get more rest, so I hadn't bothered to go again when the other symptoms appeared, because I didn't think he would listen this time either.

Sasha thought about my list of woes and suggested that I go to see Sarah, someone who had helped her during a difficult period in her own life. She told me that Sarah was a Craniosacral Therapist and an Alexander teacher, but I had barely heard of the Alexander Technique, let alone Craniosacral Therapy and thought that it all sounded a bit out of my comfort zone. Unlike Sasha I haven't had much experience of complementary therapies, apart from an occasional massage and a one-off visit to an Osteopath when I had had a bad back. I was a bit sceptical about how much complementary medicine could help. What I really needed, I thought longingly, was a good night's sleep, some space to gather my thoughts, a long holiday and if not a different family, then the same family with extras like thoughtfulness and tidiness. Sasha had told me a little about what the session involved, but I wasn't entirely convinced that a woman who I had never met putting her hands on me was going to change anything. However, Sasha was insistent that it might help, so I thought I would give it a go if only to please her. As she said, what harm could there be? The worst that might happen was that I had a pleasant hour away from home and childcare. So here I was and not terribly sure why.

I warmed to Sarah immediately, though, first because I liked her calm, unhurried attitude and because she took the time to put me at my ease, and didn't go straight into the treatment. We sat quietly as she took my address and other details, and there seemed to be no rush to get on with things. I found her voice very soothing, and began to relax, but just as I began to feel better, I remembered that I hadn't asked Sasha whether I would have to take my clothes off. I tried desperately to think if I had shaved my legs recently, and whether I had my newer underwear on or the old, grey, washed-out stuff. As often happens, I had left the house in a panic and not thought ahead. I felt my anxiety building again and wondered miserably why I had come.

Sarah said she wanted to take some more notes before we began, so I was, thankfully, able to defer that problem for a little while longer. My breathing slowly came back to normal, my fidgeting gradually decreased and I was able to take a better look at her. She appeared to be somewhere in her fifties, with short blonde hair and a warm, friendly attitude. She wasn't wearing a white coat as the Osteopath had done, just ordinary clothes, quite smart and youthful. She asked why I had come and left me to answer in my own time. Even though I was feeling more comfortable by now, my mind went completely blank at this point, and I couldn't think why on earth I was there. It seemed so unlikely that she could help me to feel less tired and stressed. All I really wanted to do was curl up in that big squashy chair and go to sleep. My head had started aching a lot, and I couldn't focus my thoughts properly. I mumbled something about needing some time away from my home life and not feeling all that well, but that I didn't think that there was anything too much wrong with me apart from exhaustion. It felt too confusing to have to go through the disconnected things that had been going wrong with my body recently, and I wasn't sure if moods and anxieties were part of her remit. When she asked me what my symptoms were, what worried me about them and when they had started, I really didn't know where to begin or what to include.

If I'm honest, I started to notice that something was wrong when I got flu a few years ago. I couldn't shake it off and just when I began to feel better it would come back. It seemed to go on for ages but perhaps it was only a couple of weeks. Since then I don't think I have ever really felt 'right'. I always seem to be irritable with the children and criticising or picking fights with Nigel. I feel that I don't have enough time, and if I do have a small window for myself I don't know what to do with it. Life seems to be a daily round of getting the children ready for school, clearing up after them, cajoling them into doing their homework and not killing themselves or each other, shopping, cooking, washing, etc. etc. I had thought that when the youngest went to school I would have more time for myself, but I just don't seem to have the energy to be interested in anything these days. I used to work for a small publisher, have always loved reading and once secretly wanted to be a writer but I no longer read anything beyond glancing at the Metro or the Evening Standard. I can't concentrate and it all seems so meaningless.

Things got considerably worse when I developed stomach problems. I began to have cramps and found myself becoming sensitive to various foods. Sometimes there are times when I think that it has gone away, but it keeps coming back, particularly when I am more cross or stressed than usual. Some days it feels as if there is nothing I can eat at all without my stomach reacting. Recently, and on top of everything else, I have started to have really bad insomnia. Despite the fact that I am so bone-chillingly tired, I will often be awake most of the night, pacing around the house trying to stop thoughts racing through my head. Sometimes I don't sleep at all, but just constantly replay stupid events of the day until I get so tired and frustrated at not being able to sleep that I want to scream.

I didn't tell Sarah all of this because I didn't want to seem too much of a basket case. Instead I simply told her again that I was feeling run down and had difficulty sleeping. I was a bit embarrassed to say more than that as I didn't really know enough about what she did to gauge what was relevant. Anyway, I was too exhausted to go through it all with her. I was worried it might all sound too self-absorbed and self-pitying, and I was also afraid that if she asked me any more questions I might start crying.

Sarah must have guessed how I was feeling because she just put down her pen and suggested that I lie down on the treatment table, saying that she didn't really need to know any more at this time. I was very relieved when she said, 'You don't need to take anything off, it all stays on.' She covered me with a warm blanket, tucked it up around me, and asked if I was comfortable. She sat herself down on a stool and waited for a minute or two. Then she asked me to relax and begin to feel my body on the table. I didn't really know what she meant by that, my brain was still in a fog, and I hoped she wasn't going to ask me too many more questions about what I was feeling. I didn't think I would know how to reply if she did. I found myself wanting to say something clever to please her and earn some brownie points by giving the right answer. But what was the right answer? I had no idea.

She held my head very gently between her hands and asked me to notice my feet and legs, then my hip joints and pelvis. It was all very odd; she didn't actually do anything other than hold my head, but gradually I became aware of the weight of my body as I was lying there. She guided my attention slowly from my pelvis up to my head and as she did so I realised that I had never really paid any attention to what my *body* was actually feeling unless it was in pain or discomfort. For quite some time as we were going through this process, I couldn't stop my thoughts from churning around and irritatingly I kept losing track of what she was saying. In an attempt to divert my own attention I looked around the room, at least the parts of it that I could see from where I was lying. It was a medium-sized room, painted soft white and with a few abstract pictures on the wall. I couldn't see them very well from where I was, but the colours were cool and restful, and they were similar to the colours that Sarah was wearing. She seemed to fit well into her room, and it reflected her personality. Her hands were warm and soothing like her voice and gradually I found myself letting go. Eventually I closed my eyes.

After a time, Sarah moved her stool and put one hand under the top of my back and another under my stomach. She still didn't seem to be doing anything and I remember thinking that although this felt quite nice and comforting, it was all a bit of a waste of time. The next thing I was aware of was waking up after what seemed like the deepest sleep I had had for ages. I thought I must have been out for hours, but Sarah said it was only about 40 minutes. I couldn't believe how calm and peaceful I was, and the thought floated through my head that she had given me my body back. At least that was the only way I could find to describe it. It was a lovely feeling, but I couldn't get over the fact that she hadn't actually *done* anything. I noticed that for the first time in ages my headache had gone. I had become so used to having low-level pain in the background that I hadn't even thought about mentioning it until now.

I got off the table and sat down in the chair again and asked Sarah what she had done to get rid of my headache and make me feel so relaxed. She smiled and said that she had just 'listened to my body', an answer I found a bit annoying and vague. I thought she must have done *something* to send me off to sleep like that, even if I couldn't feel anything. She said that she had noticed that my body was extremely tired (I could have told her that) and that I needed to start paying some attention to myself before I developed more serious symptoms. She suggested having some regular sessions, with a review after about six, and explained that it was something like having psychotherapy except that it worked through the body. We apparently needed some time to get know each other in order to allow the work to develop and for changes to occur. I was pleased that I wasn't expected to think or talk or explain what I had felt, as the last place I wanted to be was back in my revolving thoughts. In fact it was such a relief to be able to just sit quietly without having to respond to anyone and I was rather dreading having to go back home.

I agreed to see her next week, and even if I just spend the next appointment in that lovely deep sleep again, it will definitely be worth the fee. I certainly don't get *that* quality of sleep very often. I'll try to be on time for the next session as well, because I don't want to feel as stressed as I did today. I need to have as much time as possible to enjoy that peaceful space and not waste it by being wound up.

## Sarah's Story

Anna came into the room like a whirlwind at our first meeting. She was out of breath and red in the face and looked as if she had been running. She was 20 minutes late and very apologetic. I wondered briefly if her lateness was a habit or whether she had just not worked out the journey yet. I am always pretty punctual, so lateness is something that interests me. Was Anna a serial latecomer or was this just a one off? Time would tell. I didn't have a client afterwards, so I could run over if necessary, but I didn't want to establish a precedent. I usually find it best to establish boundaries early on so that people don't feel resentful later, but 40 minutes is not long enough to take a case history and give a treatment, and I could see she was in a bit of a state. I decided to play it by ear.

I showed Anna to a chair and invited her to make herself comfortable while I took a few notes. I wanted to slow things down a bit and let her recover from her journey, so my first questions were quite general. I asked whether she knew anything about Craniosacral Therapy or Alexander Technique, and she replied that she had never had this kind of treatment before and had no idea what it might involve. I explained that I worked with both disciplines, and that although there was a different emphasis to each, essentially I would be putting my hands gently on her body and trying to find areas where she was holding unnecessary tension. As we talked, I had a chance to observe her a little. Physically she was slight and wiry. She wore her long, dark hair caught up in an untidy knot at the back of her head. She gave the impression of having dressed in a hurry that morning. Her face was small with large, wide-set, anxious eyes, and she looked confused as she tried to find answers to my questions. Listening to her voice, I began to have a strange feeling that I had met her somewhere before, but I knew that I definitely hadn't. Maybe she reminded me of someone.

Anna seemed to be struggling to take on board what I was saying, and her movements were jumpy. Suddenly she appeared to remember something, and started rummaging in her bag, accidentally turning the contents out onto the floor. She found her tissues and switched off her mobile, apologising frantically for being so clumsy. I began to feel very sorry for her; she appeared so inept. While she was fishing around in her bag, I had the opportunity to watch her more closely. She was obviously in a state of high stimulation, very red faced and breathing fast. I realised I needed to keep an eye on my own breathing, which wanted to accelerate to keep pace with hers. It was hard work to slow myself down, so I concentrated on that while she continued to fidget. When she had finished picking up her things and had eventually settled herself back in the chair I saw that she was sitting in a crumpled heap, very awkward and twisted up. It all looked very uncomfortable, and I saw in her body a familiar mixture of extreme tension and collapse.

After a while when she was breathing more easily, I began to try to find out why she had come. She stared at me for a moment, as if she had no idea how to answer my question. Eventually she said that her friend Sasha, a long-term client of mine, had suggested she come to see me because she hadn't been feeling well for some time. She thought perhaps she was just run down, but found it hard to relax and get to sleep, even though she was really tired. From time to time she had stomach cramps and indigestion, and often felt bloated. As she spoke I noticed that she played all her symptoms down, as if they were of little importance. I asked whether she had seen her GP about any of this but she said that she hadn't wanted to trouble him since it was all rather vague and might be a waste of his time. She said she didn't want to waste my time either, she was probably just making a fuss, but everything about her was telling me a different story. She looked totally exhausted, with bags under her eyes and the beginnings of a cold sore at the corner of her mouth. I learned that she would be 41 this year, was married and had three children of varying ages. I jotted down this information along with my observations, but getting any further information out of Anna was a bit like pulling teeth. She seemed too tired to answer.

Because I could see she was exhausted and was finding it difficult to focus, I decided to get her straight onto the couch rather than asking any more questions. Her lack of response didn't feel deliberately obstructive, but more an inability to connect either with herself or her symptoms. I wondered if she would be any more forthcoming when she was lying down, because at times she seemed to want to avoid looking me directly in the eye. I've noticed before that when clients are very stressed or traumatised eye contact can be quite challenging and that not having to engage directly can offer some form of protection. I asked if she would like to lie down, and after I had reassured her that she didn't need to take her clothes off, I offered her a blanket and began the treatment. She asked nervously if she would be all right to drive after the treatment, as she had to pick up her children from school. I told her that ideally she should rest for a little while, but that she should be fine. I then suggested that she start to notice what her body was feeling as she was lying on my treatment table.

Before I tried to listen more closely to Anna's body I needed to be aware of my own state, my feet on the ground and the room around me. She was all coiled and held, even though she lay reasonably flat on my table. I was finding it quite hard not to get caught up in her contagious nervous energy and I noticed my own thoughts flowing faster than normal. I could see strong cords of tension in Anna's neck and shoulders. It was as if she was trying to take up as little space as possible, just as she had done in the chair earlier. She was obviously anxious to see how this mysterious treatment would unfold, and her body was reflecting this. She looked jittery and on the verge of bolting, with all of her senses on high alert.

I wasn't sure where to start, but since she appeared to be completely disconnected and distanced from herself in general, I decided the first thing to do would be to begin by bringing her into contact with her own body. My heart went out to her because I remembered only too clearly feeling like that myself. I know what it is like to be uncomfortable in your own skin. It had been a long time ago, but I could still remember the misery and discomfort of those days. I wondered for a moment if the reason Anna had seemed familiar was because I was reminded of an earlier version of myself.

Her anxiety was so insistent that it was drowning out everything else and probably consuming an enormous amount of her resources. It seemed the first and most obvious thing to tackle before we could start to see what was underneath. The symptoms that Anna had described might well come under the umbrella of 'stress', but it was too early to tell. She certainly seemed to have all the signs of someone whose energy levels were almost completely depleted, but for the moment I did not know why. If this was Anna's habitual state, I wasn't surprised that she was so run down. I began by taking her through some simple ways of coming into contact with her body, although I knew that at first she would probably be unable to do this easily.

I cupped her head in my hands, remembering to stay aware of myself and my breathing. I asked Anna to notice her own breath, the movement of her ribs gently expanding and contracting and the sensation of air coming and going through her nose. Next I asked her to imagine lying on a beach and to feel the impression her body would make in the sand. Could she be aware of the weight of her pelvis, her lower back, her arms and her legs, all settling into the sand and leaving their mark? Very slowly I guided her attention through her body, all the while keeping my hands around her head. Everything seemed very disharmonious and scattered, but gradually I noticed through my fingers a slight slowing down of her nervous system. Her body felt simultaneously exhausted and very tightly held in various places, and there was a strong sense that, despite her extreme tension, she wasn't really present at all, but floating somewhere above the couch. I noticed that I immediately wanted to analyse and explain this, but reminded myself to settle down and wait, trusting that if I could be quiet enough something else might have a chance to emerge.

This part of a treatment is a bit like waiting for the birds to begin singing again after they have been disturbed; nothing happens until a particular quality of silence and safety have returned. As I sat quietly, waiting, I began to be aware of a split between the upper and lower halves of her body and of the fact that there were various centres around which everything seemed to be continuously revolving.

I found my hands drawn to make contact behind her shoulder blades and under her solar plexus. These two areas seemed most in need of attention. After a time I felt her breathing change and become more even. I could feel that she hadn't actually fallen asleep and knew that she was in that halfway point between consciousness and unconsciousness where the body will often begin to respond. This extraordinary state of almost lucid dreaming is characteristic of Craniosacral Therapy and experienced by most clients at some point during a course of treatments. Anna's whole body became softer and began to feel more expansive and joined up. Some of the tight knots began to release. There was obviously a long way to go but I was pleased to know she was responding to my touch, and I felt hopeful that we could work together successfully. Perhaps next time we could start to look at some of the reasons behind her exhaustion and start to piece together her background story.

I finished the session by taking my hands away from her head and stepped back to give her time to sit up and look around. I was curious to find out how she was feeling and what she had made of the treatment. Her first question was a familiar one. What had I found, and what did I do? Although I was more concerned to hear what she had thought and felt, I gave her a simple answer. I could see that she had no frame of reference for this work and so I just said that I had listened to her body and that I could tell that her energy was severely depleted. I suggested that she take this seriously, that symptoms like hers were not necessarily random events but signs that she needed to take more care of herself and perhaps explore their deeper causes. I was pretty sure that it would take some time for her to begin to appreciate the benefit of the therapy so I told her that I would recommend seeing her weekly for a while but that we should have a review after six sessions to make sure that things were moving in the right direction.

I was glad that she agreed to commit to more sessions over the next few months because that would give us time to get to the bottom of things. As I had minimal case notes I had very little idea of Anna's history but I had a suspicion that there was more going on than just tiredness. Privately, I felt that it might take some time, depending on her response both to me and to the work. Working in this way is such an individual process and can move in so many different directions that it is hard to tell after one session where things will end up. I was interested in Anna though, and wanted to continue to work with her. I could already feel that we had a lot of life experiences in common and I felt I could help her.

## Our Story

### LIZ AND DAŠKA

When someone comes in for a treatment, it is a whole person who enters the room and not just a sore shoulder or leg or a bad back. If we are only concerned with the relief of pain, and not the relationship of the sore back to the body as a whole, then we are looking to cure, not to heal. Many questions come to mind when meeting someone with a bad back. Why is her back aching and not her head? Why is this person suffering and what is it that really troubles her? Why has she chosen her back to bear her pain? By concentrating solely on 'fixing' her back, we may be ignoring a deeper malaise that is struggling to come to the surface. If we fixate on the idea of alleviating pain from one area alone, we are almost certainly missing the larger picture and could be changing things for the worse and not the better. Real healing takes place in an atmosphere of mutual inquiry.

### DAŠKA

In Chapter One we look at a first session and how it might play out in real life. As a practitioner I'm often nervous during the early stages of a treatment programme because naturally I very much want it to be a success. I used to feel very insecure about my work, and 20 years later those same feelings can still surface unexpectedly, although I have now learned not to pay them too much attention. Things can get difficult if I find myself resonating either with my client's stories or with their reactions to those stories. Since I have struggled with aspects of this in my own work, we decided to use my experience to show the reality of how a practitioner might feel in practice.

First sessions are interesting but often inconclusive. There are always plenty of questions. How is this relationship going to develop, and will it even get off the ground? What is this client bringing? Can I help her? I particularly notice what people tell me and what they leave out. Omissions may often mean that they have not yet made the connection between their symptoms and their lifestyle or history. The mind/body connection is usually obvious and tangible to us as practitioners, but many people see the two as entirely separate and may never have considered that the way that they stand or sit may be one of the causes of their depression as well as their backache. Most symptoms are a result of a number of disparate factors, which leads to confusion. While not every twinge has a deep psychological meaning, our bodies do register everything they have ever experienced and store our memories and emotions along with our physical shapes. Initially, I try to establish a sense of safety and a space where clients can start to feel at home and begin to trust me and the process. In any developing relationship it takes time to get to know one another and for confidence to grow. If the client is new to this type of work, it can be truly surprising to her to find that the results can extend beyond the merely physical. Like Anna, I too originally came to bodywork with no idea of what my body was trying to tell me.

As Joseph Campbell has pointed out,[3] the myths of the Hero's Journey often follow the same pattern: the hero or heroine has come to an impasse where all their old ways of being in the world no longer seem to be working. Mythical stories generally begin with the hero experiencing a separation from all the familiar patterns of life. The point of no return propels the protagonist into a new situation where she is forced into sinking or swimming. After a lengthy and intense period of journeying, either internally or externally, there is the return to the world with new skills.

---

3    Campbell, J. (ed.) (1949/1973) *The Hero with a Thousand Faces*. Princeton, NJ: Princeton University Press.

In Anna's story, as it was for me, her body and psyche are the catalyst for the start of this adventure, they are 'breaking down' and no longer able to contain the turmoil of her mind and emotions. Her body has become like the Waste Land of the Fisher King in the old Grail legend, and may well continue to throw up increasingly awkward symptoms compelling her either to face her situation or succumb to it. In the legend we encounter the medieval hero Perceval and see his progression from 'innocent fool' into responsibility and full consciousness. Like many heroes, Perceval's true heritage has been hidden from him and he grows knowing nothing of his 'noble' birth. Perceval's mother has lost her husband and his three older brothers to wars and the excessively patriarchal chivalric code of the time. In order to save her last son from this fate she hides him from the court, keeping him innocent and dressing him in 'homespun' cloth. One of the many themes of this great legend is the story of the awakening of Perceval's consciousness. He must leave his mother and his beginnings and grow up, not just into a man but also to assume his heritage and rightful position in life. His adventures lead him to the magical castle of the Fisher King. The King has been wounded and is unable to heal, and his kingdom has become the Waste Land. The story is an allegory of the dissociation of spirit from nature, or mind from body. In the myth, the King can only be healed and the Waste Land restored to fertility by the spontaneous compassion of an innocent. Perceval was such a compassionate innocent but his upbringing initially prevented him from asking the healing question. He was unable to heal the King until he had matured sufficiently and it would not be until he returned in middle age after countless adventures that he stumbled once more on the castle and was able at last to reconcile his distorted upbringing with the lessons subsequently learned.

We use this story particularly because it shows that an overwhelming feminine function could be just as harmful as an overarching masculine function. Perceval's task is to learn to reconcile these two opposites in himself.

## LIZ

Anna's session with Sarah is fairly typical of a first session with someone who has had little experience of complementary therapies. Anna is flustered, wound up and dissociated. She has made herself late for her appointment and is unable to settle. Sarah's calmness is attractive because it is such a contrast to how she is feeling herself, but there is a potential for it to be intimidating or even shaming. It's easy for us to forget how uncomfortable the first session can be for someone who is feeling this desperate and unhappy. Anna's mind goes blank when she tries to answer Sarah's questions. The overwhelming tiredness and anxiety that she is experiencing mean that she downplays her symptoms, not wishing to feel under further pressure. Once on the couch she can relax more, but she doesn't quite know how to behave in this situation. Sarah has not explained much about the therapy, what she does or how it works, so Anna is in the dark and searching for ways in which to connect.

It's possible that Sarah feels that giving Anna a detailed, technical description of the therapy is too much for her to absorb so soon or may not even be appropriate. Anna is quite sceptical and will need more proof that something is helping before she is ready to comprehend her own role in the process. At the moment she just needs to be looked after, and Sarah is wisely not giving her too much to digest for the moment. Sarah also decides not to take a full case history in this first session and this seems a good decision. Anna is stressed, and questioning her is only making things worse. We would normally take a full case history before beginning treatment, but there are times when it seems more appropriate to allow the client's story to emerge over a number of sessions. In a situation like this, intuition is more useful than words. Anna's physical state and the way that Sarah finds herself responding tell her far more than anything Anna could say at this point. By noticing her appearance, her body language, the tone of her voice and her own strong response to the distress, Sarah is listening in a way that will give her a fuller picture without asking questions. She can fill in the gaps in future sessions. It is very easy to make case-history taking into a meaningless ritual without considering why you need that information and how it may be helpful. It can be easy to be led astray by what a client may tell you at the beginning of a course of treatments; at this stage Anna is not in a place where she is able to connect either with herself or her symptoms.

I have often found that the most illuminating thing a client says is just as she is about to leave. So many times someone has turned as they are about to open the door and said 'By the way…'!

# CHAPTER TWO

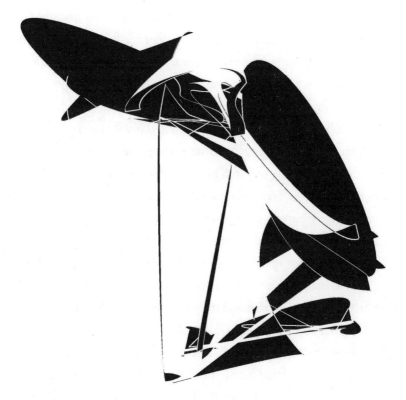

# FEELING THE WAY

## Anna's Story

I'm not at all sure what I hoped for from my first treatment with Sarah. Not much really, I think my mild scepticism got in the way of any real expectations. I admit I was surprised at how remarkably calm and peaceful I felt after the session. Of course it didn't last. I got home and was almost instantly overwhelmed by the demands of the household and the whole daily round of mindless tasks that just had to be done. I did notice, however, that I slept really deeply for a long time on the night after the session and woke feeling rested. Other than that I didn't see any lasting difference except that possibly I didn't feel quite so anxious. My insomnia was much as it had been before. I still felt exhausted and on edge and my stomach continued to trouble me. From time to time during the following week, I found myself thinking of Sarah and remembering the extraordinary space and calm that I had experienced, but as the week went on it all seemed to have happened in another lifetime. I did realise, though, that I was really looking forward to the next session.

I made a major effort to be on time for my next appointment. Sarah welcomed me in with a friendly smile that made me feel instantly at home and showed me to the usual chair. I had thought this time that she would go straight ahead with the treatment, and quite honestly all I wanted to do was get on the couch and fall asleep. The previous night I had hardly slept a wink, and the morning chaos with the children had been really difficult to handle. Instead Sarah sat down and asked how I had been and what if anything I had noticed since we last met. I couldn't think of anything significant to say except that I had slept better for that one night, and maybe a little better on the following nights, but last night had been awful. She asked about my headaches and I realised that I hadn't noticed any since our last session. I wasn't sure what else she expected me to say. Nothing much seemed to have happened, and as I said all I really wanted to do was to get onto the table again and for her to start the session. Sarah said that at this stage she hadn't expected major changes but that she thought the fact that I had experienced some better sleep and that the headaches had improved was a sign that I was responding to the treatment. I found this reassuring, but did begin to wonder how long she thought it would be before I felt really better and if indeed I was going to at all.

I had phoned Sasha for a chat during the week. I wanted to know more about her experience. Had Sarah worked in the same way with her, what was she doing when she put her hands on and why was the therapy so relaxing? I was curious that such a light touch could send you off to sleep so quickly and leave you feeling amazing, if only temporarily. I told her I really liked Sarah, and had warmed to her immediately, but I didn't yet know if she could help me, because I didn't understand what she was doing. Sasha said that to begin with she had found it all a bit mysterious. Like me she had been unconvinced after her first session. She went on to say that I shouldn't give up too quickly; it was important to give it a chance. She had needed quite a few sessions before she felt better. I heard what she was saying, but I was secretly praying that it wouldn't take me as long as that. I wanted to feel better as quickly as possible. I didn't know if I could take these feelings of illness and tiredness for much longer, certainly not if it was going to take weeks or months. I had been shocked to see the contrast between how I had felt after the treatment and the way I have become used to feeling day to day.

Perhaps noticing that I was looking a bit distracted, Sarah said that she had asked enough questions for the moment and invited me to get on the couch. When she was certain I was comfortable, she sat and talked quietly to me for a few moments before making contact. She said she wanted to be sure I was ready before we started the treatment. Apparently it takes a while to form a working relationship with a client, and a mutual understanding and trust only develop over time. It is like making a new friend. You have to establish a common language, and this can only evolve gradually. Taking a few minutes to get used to each other's presence allows a treatment to develop in a natural and organic way. I was perfectly happy just lying down, so I said it was fine.

After a few moments Sarah checked that I was ready to begin, but before she settled into the session she said she could see that the way that I was lying looked unnaturally tight, and she would like to be able to teach me how to release before continuing. She asked me to notice my neck and shoulders and see if I could allow them to release into her hands. I wasn't sure how to do this, but she suggested that I tighten them more and then let go, and that seemed to work. She then asked me to add an awareness of the sensation of my pelvis on the table and to begin to think about my backbone as one piece from the sacrum right up to my neck. She told me that my spine actually began in the middle of my head behind my nose and that I could start to help myself by thinking of space in my body, in my neck and at the top of my spine. This all sounded very nice, although I don't think I quite got the bit about space, but something must have worked because I was gradually aware of my whole back softening and expanding and coming into contact with the table. Sarah moved her hands to my right shoulder and it was only when she touched it that I realised how much tension I was holding. It was aching and the pain seemed to go right up the side of my neck. What was odd was that she didn't do anything apart from hold the shoulder while asking me to notice my lower back. Again the noticing thing was difficult, but bit by bit I felt the whole of my upper back opening out into her hands and slowly melting. Although this was a pleasant feeling overall, I was surprised to discover that as well as feeling relaxed I was also uneasy, and I found myself continually tightening up again without knowing why. It was hard to stay with the feeling of softness and melting when my body was fighting against it. More frustrating and confusing was a feeling of panic, which I didn't understand or recognise. Surely what I wanted was to feel relief from tightness, but something was subconsciously preventing me from doing so.

Sarah must have picked up that I was struggling with this, and she started to talk about how the way we think and hold ourselves affects us both physically and emotionally. I hadn't thought about it like that before. She asked me to go back to tightening my neck and shoulders and to notice how that made me feel, and then to release and notice again. I found that the tightening made me feel safe but at the same time anxious and tense. The feelings were really familiar, and I realised that this was my usual state of being. She said that what was important was not that there was any right or wrong way to be but that it might be helpful for me to start to notice what was happening.

After a while, Sarah said that she would now allow the work to move into a quieter, more cranial space. She put one hand under the middle of my back and the other under my lower back and sat quietly. I was aware of the heat of her hands and a warmth spreading through my whole body and I closed my eyes. I found I really liked Sarah's touch. It was comforting and gave me a sense of everything being okay. This sense of security allowed me to drift away to a different level. It was a very odd sensation because I could hear noises like the birds outside and the distant sounds of the city and yet it was as if I was deeply asleep. I don't remember being so relaxed in my whole life. During this period, thoughts and images streamed through my mind without any sense or meaning. At one point I became aware of a distinct but still dreamlike sensation that I was very young again, around the age of six or seven. I had the strangest feeling in the pit of my stomach, familiar yet elusive, which I struggled to pin down. The more I tried, the more it escaped me. I couldn't seem to catch it full on. The only way I can describe it is like seeing something from the corner of my eye. After a while the impression disappeared, and although I thought about mentioning it to Sarah, I couldn't find the words, and didn't really want to disturb the bubble of stillness in which we were enclosed. Momentarily I had felt a bit uncomfortable, but I couldn't work out where it had come from, so I dismissed it and settled back into that magically quiet space.

Much too quickly, the session was over. Reluctantly, I came back to the present moment and sat up on the couch, still feeling very drowsy and heavy. I was dying to know what Sarah had felt during the treatment, so I asked her to tell me. She said that she had felt tension in lots of areas of my body and that she thought she had noticed a particularly knotted area around the solar plexus. She asked me what I had felt and I started to try to explain the odd feeling I had experienced in the pit of my stomach. By this time it was getting quite vague and I no longer felt so connected to it, so I just said that I had felt a bit strange. She seemed okay with this explanation, so I pulled myself together, we confirmed next week's appointment time and I went off to face the world.

## Sarah's Story

I was curious to know what Anna had made of the treatment and wondered whether any of the effects had lasted or if her body had tightened up again. Craniosacral Therapy can deepen and develop during the days after a session, but the effects need to build up over several sessions, and so I wasn't really expecting any significant changes after just one meeting.

For her second session a week later, Anna arrived punctually. She was more confident this time, less hesitant and nervous than before. I asked how she had felt after the last session, and she said that not much had changed. On the night of the treatment she had slept much better and for a short while afterwards had felt very relaxed. Since then, however, she had not been sleeping well and over the past week her insomnia had got progressively worse. Her stomach problems, too, were much the same. I told her that I wasn't particularly concerned that there hadn't been an immediate improvement in her symptoms because I suspected that they had taken quite a long time to build up. I thought privately that they may have become very much part of a habitual pattern and might take some time to shift. I just hoped that she would be able to develop enough patience and trust to give the work time to progress. I was fairly sure that stress and tension were major factors, if not the main cause of her symptoms. If that was the case then, in the long term, helping her to make a connection between mind and body and teaching her some simple methods of relieving tension would be the most effective treatment.

At the very end of our last meeting Anna had mentioned that she sometimes suffered from quite bad recurrent headaches, so I asked her how they had been.

'It's odd,' she said, 'but I hadn't even noticed that I haven't had a headache this week. Perhaps the weather has changed or something?'

I smiled inwardly as she said this because it is so familiar. At the beginning clients are often very reluctant to credit the therapy for any change in their symptoms. Because they don't yet understand how Craniosacral Therapy works, they would much rather look to something more tangible for an answer. I decided not to say anything though, because I didn't know yet what was causing any of her symptoms.

I saw that Anna didn't really want to talk much more and decided to get her straight onto the table again without further questioning. She looked as if she was longing to lie down and said that she had really been looking forward to the session. I could see that the effort of climbing onto the couch caused her to contract her shoulders and neck and tighten her jaw. I thought this might be a good moment to show her how she could lie more comfortably and feel more at ease with herself. It would be empowering for her to start to learn how to release her own tension. Depression can give you the feeling that everything is out of control and you are unable to change anything, and I wondered if Anna was depressed and heading towards the state that I had been in before I had discovered bodywork. I found myself resonating strongly with her discomfort.

Last time I had suggested that Anna start to notice the amount of muscular tension that she was holding in her neck and shoulders, and today I asked her if she could begin to release it while she was lying on the table. She seemed to enjoy this part of the treatment, noticing how much difference small changes in her thinking and positioning made to her overall sense of relaxation and well-being. She commented at one moment that she couldn't feel me doing anything, so could not understand how her shoulders felt so much wider and softer. I wasn't surprised to notice that she slowly and almost imperceptibly tightened up again when I had moved to another part of her body, although her muscle contraction wasn't quite so exaggerated overall. It is an odd feeling to have a stranger rearrange your body and any change in position inevitably makes you feel different and awkward. I explained to Anna that I believe the way we feel can sometimes be caused by the way that we carry ourselves. As body language is so much easier to read in others than it is to recognise in ourselves, she was probably unaware how much the constraint in her own body had been affecting her. I asked her to notice over the next week how she felt physically when she was either happy or sad. How was she emotionally when she tightened her neck? I could see that Anna hadn't thought in these terms before and that I had planted a seed that we would be able to explore in future sessions.

I spent some time gradually encouraging a sense of ease and space in her body before moving into the quieter and more still work of Craniosacral Therapy. I held Anna's feet beneath her ankles, and waited for us both to drop into a deeper place.

As I began to connect more deeply with Anna, I became aware of the quality of energy flowing through her body and subtle changes in her breathing. I noticed once again the paradoxical feelings of restriction and apathy I had felt last week. It was becoming increasingly obvious to me that her condition had developed over a long period of time and was not solely related to her current situation. However, I was pleased to see that Anna had now closed her eyes and appeared to be responding to the treatment more readily than she had done before. Her hands were resting lightly on her chest, and the line of her jaw had softened. I moved to put one hand on Anna's stomach and the other under her back. There was a feeling of peace in the room, a sense of timelessness.

I stayed with my contact until the hour was up and it felt as if we were ready for the session to come to an end. Anna got up slowly from the couch, yawning and stretching as she did so. When she was bending to put on her shoes, she looked up and asked what I had felt and I told her about the tension that I had found in her solar plexus. It had seemed to me both tight and exposed. I was worried that being so open and unprotected there meant that she might be too vulnerable to meet the outside world without more robust boundaries. I didn't say any of this because I wasn't sure yet that it was accurate and I didn't want to alarm her. This work is very individual and it was too early to evaluate how far Anna wanted to explore.

Anna had arrived for both sessions so anxious and in need of treatment that I had put her straight onto the table. Normally I would take a comprehensive case history at the beginning of a series of treatments but for some reason I thought that she would benefit more from plunging straight in. It would help me now to hear her story and how the patterns of her life have unfolded, since the choices that we all make as a result of our circumstances have such an impact on our future. I was beginning to see that much of her past experience was deeply embedded in her system and I wanted to find out more about her. We said goodbye and arranged to meet at the same time the following week. I found myself looking forward to seeing Anna again and hoped we had made some progress.

## Our Story

### LIZ AND DAŠKA

This book has been through many stages, changing shape and shifting constantly as it has evolved. Like Anna and Sarah, we found that before we were able to work together we had to get to know each other and our respective strengths and weaknesses. We also discovered many things about ourselves; this is version six of this section and we are still learning. We called this chapter 'Feeling the Way' because it shows how our characters negotiate their developing therapeutic relationship and at the same time describes our own experience as we wrote.

This is what Liz wrote about Sarah fairly early on:

> Sarah has had a difficult life, with plenty of stress. She has had two unsuccessful relationships, which have each produced a child. She is a single mother with the youngest son at home. Her mother is a real problem, in a care home, but very difficult and can be aggressive. Possible dementia. Her father died of cancer, and had a long and painful illness. Sarah was very involved in nursing him throughout. Sarah's siblings believe it is the younger unattached daughter who should take the brunt of the mother's care, and there is a constant battle about this, because Sarah feels she has contributed as much as she can to the care of her parents. She has never been as close to her mother as she was to her father. Sarah has suffered depression, and this led her to years of psychotherapy, so although she has no qualifications as a psychotherapist, she has a good knowledge of the work and has done several counsellor trainings. She was perhaps led into the therapy field by her own need to rescue, with which she continues to struggle. Because of her own experience of depression and its cyclical nature, she tends to specialise in this and stress conditions in her work and has been very successful in helping her clients. However, she has had problems in the past with clients who have become very attached to her, and vice versa, and this is another of her learning curves.

Essentially, not much has changed. In our story Sarah connects instantly with Anna because she feels that she recognises something that is very familiar and appealing, and is starting to find it hard to separate her own emotions and sensations. We show her being worried that she sees something of herself in Anna and her struggles. She has taken minimal case notes and has no real idea what is causing Anna's problems so it's very important that she doesn't jump to conclusions, impose her own story and lose the wood for the trees. We have found while writing that it has also been hard for us to keep hold of the larger picture whilst immersing ourselves in the detail. It has been helpful to work together so that both ends of the spectrum are equally held.

Sarah picks up that Anna's muscles are unusually tight. This could signal unexpressed emotional components of which she is unaware. Emotions and thoughts are experienced in the body and disturbances at any level are reflected on all planes. If locked in for any length of time, suppressed feelings can demand to be heard and can manifest as physical problems. In our work we frequently come across symptoms that seem to have no physiological cause. They could be described as psychosomatic, a word that has some negative connotations. The word is derived from the ancient Greek words 'Psyche' meaning of the soul and 'Soma' meaning of the body. From our perspective as bodyworkers, we are baffled that in our culture this connection is still so often unrecognised. Where it is seen, it is perceived as somehow less significant than conditions with physical origins. Illness usually has more than one cause, and it is really surprising to us that the mind's effect on the body is still so poorly understood. In Craniosacral Therapy we are particularly well placed to work with issues like these since we hope to help unite mind and body through the medium of touch.

### LIZ

Touch gives us our very earliest contact with the world outside our skin. It tells us where our body ends and space begins. From five weeks a foetus will begin to respond to a stimulus on the upper lip area. By birth, our whole body is responsive to touch, and we have begun to associate it with safety and the comfort of feeding and sooner or later will use it to explore the world around us.

Early experience will profoundly colour how we feel about being touched. If we have not been held when we needed holding, if feeding has been difficult or if our exploration has resulted in rejection or trauma, it can shape our responses throughout life.

In our society we rarely touch each other unless we are in a physical relationship. In fact in many situations nowadays, touching is actively discouraged. Teachers may not touch children to comfort them because of worries about inappropriate contact. Most psychotherapists avoid touching their clients in case they give a wrong message. In all forms of bodywork we have to be aware of the possibilities of evoking emotion through the intimacy of a treatment session. This can apply to both client and therapist, since both will have early experiences that may be triggered by touch.

A person who has learned to be protective of herself may find that touch, however light, feels invasive. A client who is unable to tell you how she feels about being touched, may be lying silently screaming whilst you treat her. She may not come back. I remember an elderly person who had lived alone for many years was so grateful for my contact that she broke down in tears. Young children are usually suspicious about being touched by a stranger. Some clients are difficult to treat because they stir up feelings from your past; your touch could equally and unexpectedly precipitate unwelcome feelings in them.

Touch is personal and powerful and needs to be used with respect and thought. This is especially true in a therapeutic context, where it is particularly open to misinterpretation. You might be intending to comfort, but your client might experience your contact as seductive. A supportive contact could be felt as manipulative. Even though you are making the lightest butterfly touch, to someone who is particularly sensitive, your hands may feel crushing.

As we touch another person, either directly on the skin or through the clothing, silent messages pass between us, moving into the deeper tissues of our body and its nervous systems. We learn about each other through touch. Trust can be built, experience shared and knowledge imparted through our two-way channel of communication. It is a language through which we can communicate something of ourselves to our clients and know more about them.

The importance of touch is echoed in our language, and it is no accident that we talk of being touched when we are emotionally moved. Apart from the well-known Greek story of Midas and his Golden Touch, there is the obscure but delightful Jewish myth about the angel Lailah touching the unborn child. While the infant grows in the womb, Lailah places a lighted candle at her head so the child can see from one end of the world to the other. The angel also teaches the entire Torah, as well as the history of her soul and her ultimate destiny. Then, just before birth, the light is extinguished and the angel calls the child into the world. At the instant of birth, Lailah lightly touches her finger on the child's upper lip, as if to say 'Shh', and she forgets everything learned in the womb. It's said that the purpose of life is to recover this light and our unique destinies. The little crease, the philtrum, in our upper lip is there to remind us of the touch of the angel.

### LIZ AND DAŠKA

As a useful lens though which to illustrate the transitions Anna, Sarah and ourselves experience throughout this book we would like to introduce the myth of Demeter and Persephone that has long fascinated us both.

It is a classic narrative of the feminine experience and an allegory of awakening consciousness. The mother/daughter relationship implicitly carries within it the remembered experience of childhood and the naivety of youth but also encompasses the future rebirth of a new self. The myth gives us the three ages of women in the figures of: Hecate, Queen of the Night, the mysterious guardian of the thresholds; Demeter, the Corn goddess of Fertility; and Persephone, her daughter, the maiden or the Kore. Their story first appeared as the Hymn to Demeter, part of the larger collection of the Homeric Hymns, and describes the abduction of Persephone by Hades, the god of the underworld.

One day Persephone is innocently gathering flowers, attracted by a spectacular narcissus. Picking the flower causes the earth to open and Hades appears in his chariot to seize her and carry her underground. Persephone screams for help but the abduction is unseen by all except the sun god Helios. Her mother, Demeter, distraught at the loss of her daughter, wanders the earth for nine days without eating, drinking or washing, trying to find her. On the tenth day the ancient goddess Hecate reveals that she had heard Persephone being abducted; together they approach Helios and discover that Persephone has been given as a wife to Zeus's brother Hades. Helios, unsurprisingly, suggests that Demeter should be pleased, as it is an honourable match.

In her grief Demeter abandons her divine role as a goddess and instead assumes the disguise of an old woman. She travels to Eleusis where she acts as a nurse to the son of the King. She cannot resist feeding the child with 'divine' food and at night places him in the fire to make him immortal until she is discovered by the child's horrified mother. Demeter reveals herself and berates the unfortunate mother for not allowing her son to become an immortal. She demands that a temple dedicated to her is built in which she sits and mourns the loss of her daughter. Her withdrawal from life causes the crops and all new life to fail on earth. Despite entreaties from all of the gods she steadfastly refuses to allow growth; Zeus eventually retreats and orders Hades to return Persephone to her mother. Hades agrees but tricks Persephone into eating three pomegranate seeds thereby ensuring her return. Finally it is agreed that Persephone will spend three months of the year in the underworld with Hades as his queen and the rest of the time on Earth with Demeter. Hecate, as the goddess and guide through difficult transitions, would henceforth act as guide for Persephone on her journeys between the worlds.

Sarah is moving unconsciously towards a Demeter/Persephone relationship with Anna. Anna has begun to remember some uncomfortable childhood events, although at present these are also unacknowledged. Given time and further work, they may surface and need to be addressed. The third session will be interesting, because both of them will have to start a descent down the rabbit hole in order to bring this buried knowledge into consciousness.

We often seem to be given the clients that we need at the right moment in our own development. There is something synchronistic about the meeting between Anna and Sarah, which may help them both move forward. We also believe it is no coincidence that since Anna and Sarah arrived in our lives, clients both new and old have come in echoing aspects of what we were describing. At times it has been uncanny to find someone lying on your couch who is so like the imaginary character or situation you have just been writing about. Occasionally they have even used the same words. More extraordinary still has been that we have sometimes found ourselves behaving like Anna or Sarah. Whatever we were writing was continually arising for us personally, and this helped to confirm to us that we were on the right track.

# CHAPTER THREE

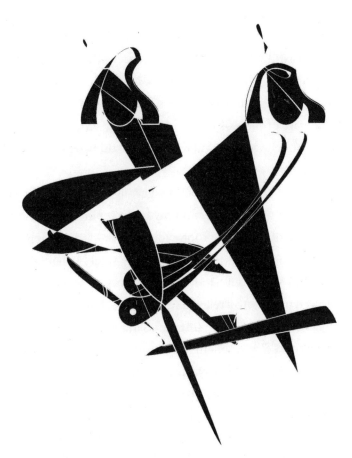

# WHERE HAVE I COME FROM?

## Anna's Story

I was back this week for my third appointment with Sarah. I can't say that I have noticed much change so far. I definitely feel very relaxed at the end of a session when I get off the couch, but it soon wears off and I'm back to feeling as depressingly overwhelmed and negative as usual. I was still intrigued about the rather odd sensations I had last time, where I had a brief memory of being quite young but was unable to remember the context. I wondered if it would happen again. One part of me was excited to see what might reveal itself, but on the whole I was reluctant to dig up anything from those days. I had enough on my plate already.

Once again I surprised myself by getting there on time. Sarah must be having a positive effect on my timekeeping if nothing else. I strode confidently into the room, looking forward to lying down for what I was beginning to think of as my weekly chance to nap without guilt. I wonder if Sarah's other clients go to sleep like me. Being allowed to fall into a relaxed semi-trance state was unexpected and enjoyable. To my disappointment Sarah asked me to sit down in the chair for a few moments because she wanted to get down some more details about my symptoms and case history.

She began by asking me some very simple questions, and I found myself unexpectedly opening up and talking about lots of things that didn't seem to connect in any way with present-day events. Once I had started, though, it all came tumbling out. She asked about the children and their ages, and I told her that Oscar is not Nigel's son. The whole dreadful story of my relationship with Steve began to come out as well. It was hard to revisit that desolate part of my life, and nowadays it's rare that I allow myself to think about it. I found myself struggling for words a lot of the time and embarrassingly close to tears. I told Sarah how alone I had felt when Steve told me he wanted nothing to do with me or my pregnancy.

He didn't want any contact with the baby and said he would pay for an abortion. I had no intention of terminating the pregnancy, and his attitude just made me more determined to go ahead. Steve was wrapped up in himself, obsessed with carving out a successful career. He was horrified at the thought of committing himself to anyone at that stage, particularly a baby. His only interest was himself and his ever-increasing status. Ironically, now, 16 years later, he is a devoted, albeit controlling, family man with two children of his own. Oscar sometimes goes to visit them, but feels out of place in Steve's perfectly designed family unit.

As I told Sarah all this, I found that I could hardly breathe, and there was a tight knot in my stomach and chest, which gave me a panicky feeling. Sarah noticed and helped me to calm down by suggesting I breathe more slowly and feel my weight on the chair. Gradually I felt better and able to continue with my story. The pregnancy was hell in so many ways. I got every symptom you can imagine: sickness, backache, depression, etc. etc. I never did become one of those glowing mothers-to-be. I was always tired and grey faced, trying to keep up with my job and my health and all the time hoping that Steve would change his mind and come back to me. By the time I got to the hospital for the delivery I realised that this wasn't going to be, but I still held a faint hope that he might come to see us or at least send a bunch of flowers. Of course, none of that happened. I went through the whole awful delivery on my own. Even my family didn't feel it necessary to give me any support, so it was just me and Oscar, trying to get through it together. Looking back I can't believe how young and naive I was.

The birth itself was a complete nightmare. Oscar was quite a big baby and took ages to arrive. In the end they had to pull him out with forceps. Afterwards I looked at him and thought he was amazing, but I was left feeling that it could all have been so much better if Steve had been there as well. Lying by myself in the hospital bed and watching all the other new fathers visiting, I was more alone than ever. I was sad for months afterwards and cried a lot of the time. Eventually I went to the doctor and he diagnosed mild postnatal depression and offered me anti-depressants, but I didn't feel like taking them. I went to see a counsellor for a while too, but that didn't help much either. I didn't like him very much; he seemed dictatorial and patronising and didn't understand at all what I was going through so I stopped seeing him.

Telling Sarah about the counsellor was interesting because it started me thinking about Sarah herself. Her approach is so different; she just listens and I don't feel judged in any way. A lot of the time she's very quiet and still, especially when she puts her hands on. I think she even closes her eyes sometimes when she's treating me, as if she too is going to sleep, but I always know she's there, and it doesn't feel as if she has drifted off. Her presence is calm and professional, and even feels quite maternal in that her hands are very warm and soothing. I don't remember my mother listening to me like Sarah does; she was always too busy with her own life to take too much notice, and she rarely touched me. My parents split up when I was little and went their own ways, which involved marrying again and giving me several stepbrothers and stepsisters.

I brought myself up as best I could. To me this became normality. I became self-reliant, but I sometimes think it might also have made me detached at times, like my mother. I wondered if Sarah has any children. I couldn't see any family photographs in the room but that didn't mean anything. I'm sure she would be a good mother. I don't think I'm such an awful mother myself, considering my background. At the beginning, Oscar and I were very close. I wonder if he sometimes resents the fact that now I've got the other two, I don't have so much time to spend with him. Perhaps what is making him so moody and uncommunicative at the moment is that he feels there is a distance between us. He's definitely quite different from the sweet, confiding little boy he used to be. The other two are finding him very hard to deal with, and so is my husband, Nigel, who tries very hard to be a good father to them all.

Recounting this story to Sarah was illuminating. I don't really talk about that part of my life to anyone, preferring to bury and hide it even from myself. I was surprised that hearing my familiar story spoken aloud seemed to give me a different perspective. I recognised how lonely and frightened I had been in those days. I don't think I had realised how severely this had affected both my physical and emotional health. I was beginning to think that my problems may have begun very much earlier than I had previously imagined. Could the roots of my present problems possibly lie in that buried period of my life?

After Sarah had finished writing down all the things I had told her she asked me to get onto the couch again. By this time I was completely exhausted. Thinking and talking about what I had gone through had really taken it out of me. I was ready for that lovely feeling of letting go to come over me. This time the session seemed to go even more quickly than before, and I can't remember where Sarah put her hands or what I thought about. I only noticed towards the end that my head wanted to roll from side to side, and I had no idea who was moving it, Sarah or me. I was left afterwards with the feeling that something had lifted, although I couldn't necessarily tell you what it was. I felt clearer in my brain, as if I had finally let go of something that had been weighing down on me for a long time.

I'm really looking forward to the next session…this one seems to have been revealing in unexpected ways.

## Sarah's Story

Before Anna arrived I decided that this time I needed to hear more of her story. In our last session I had been aware of a focus around her solar plexus. I had written that it had felt like nervous energy and confusingly appeared to be both tightly held and swirling around. There was a quality of resistance to it that had made me wonder how long it had been there and how much of an emotional component it contained. I didn't know what had caused it or what it was about, and although I felt it was important, I reminded myself to go slowly and let Anna take the lead.

I began by asking about her family and her children. She told me that her eldest son has a different father to her two other children and that the first pregnancy had been difficult for her both physically and emotionally. She had become a single mother when the baby's father had abandoned her shortly after finding out she was pregnant. Being very young, she was unprepared for the demands of motherhood. She had probably suffered from mild postnatal depression and her GP had suggested anti-depressants, but in the end she had chosen not to take them and had settled instead for an unsuccessful attempt at counselling. I could see that telling her story was deeply affecting for Anna. She was finding it difficult to get her words out, and I wanted to go over to her and give her a big hug. Instead I helped her to breathe more slowly and ground herself. After a while she continued and told me about her family background and her childhood. I was not surprised to hear that she had not had an easy upbringing. Some things were beginning to fall into place.

At present, she went on, she was dealing with the difficulties of managing a moody adolescent and the demands of her two younger children. Although she didn't say this in so many words, I picked up that her life was a balancing act and that she was tired of being the emotional lynchpin of the house. I wondered how much time she had for herself, but knowing that she was bringing up a young family I knew it would be a silly question.

I had been fairly sure that the disturbances that I had felt in her body and nervous system had much earlier roots, but now I saw that it might have been compounded by the fear and trauma of the pregnancy. I still didn't feel I had got to the bottom of what was going on with Anna but suspected that she didn't know either. I was very conscious that her story had really moved me. The connection I had felt with Anna from our first session had deepened and I realised that it was all horribly familiar. Some of it was very close to what had happened to me. I too have children from different relationships and have had little family support so I understood the difficulties that she was facing only too well. I found I too was almost in tears.

Collecting myself, I decided that she had probably told me enough and it was time to put her on the table and let her story evolve gradually as we went along. This time I found that she settled easily and I was able to connect with her fairly quickly. We were more in tune with each other now, and I felt that Anna was beginning to trust me. It takes time for clients to notice any lasting difference in their symptoms and to develop confidence in me and the work, and that is why I always encourage them to have a course of treatments. It is vital to establish a trusting relationship with each other, and I felt Anna and I were moving towards that goal.

Working at this level, security and safety are paramount; it can be so intimate and intense that people often wonder if I know what they're thinking. In the early days of my own therapy I wondered that myself. I actually don't have any idea of what is in people's minds, although I am often aware that they are thinking. I notice that the whole texture of the body changes as if all their energy and attention has rushed to the head.

One thing I do work hard at is helping people to feel secure in their own bodies as well as their minds. In one of my first Alexander Technique lessons I felt as if I was coming home to my body for the first time. This was such a remarkable experience for me that I now consciously try to invoke that profound sense of safety and homecoming in my own work. Over the years I have noticed that many of us don't actually live in our bodies. It is sad that by choosing to ignore the feeling tones of the body, we lose a huge amount of our sensory awareness.

I began the treatment by slowly organising Anna on the table, allowing her time to become more aware of her physical self and to take a breath. This part of the treatment is really important for us both. We are coming into a relationship with with each other and preparing for what might arise in this session. I was almost immediately drawn to the area just below her shoulder blades, which often holds an emotional charge. I slid one of my hands underneath her back and let my other hand support her neck. I waited and after a time asked silently what she might need. I was almost instantly conscious of her whole system slowing, becoming watchful and waiting to see what would happen. Gradually and almost imperceptibly I felt myself drop into a dreamlike space. Anna's neck began to move from side to side, rolling and releasing itself in a gentle unwinding. It seems that the restricted muscles in Anna's neck and upper thorax had taken the opportunity to untwist their tight fascial coverings. Each time her neck reached its furthest point on either side, I held it there gently until there was a softening and melting, and it was able to move on into a deeper and stronger pattern of resistance. Eventually it slowed and came to a halt.

Information appears to me in many different ways. Sometimes I am aware of a single image, and at other times I can see a whole story unfolding. From time to time I can feel sensations in my own body

WHERE HAVE I COME FROM?

or hear snatches of songs. There are also days when I feel nothing at all. Today, as I held Anna's neck, I had an image of holding a small bird with a broken wing. The bird appeared terrified and I knew that I had to keep holding it until its heart stopped beating so furiously. Later I became aware of conflicting emotions spinning around. A sense of working hard but an accompanying resentment. A desire to drop everything and run away and at the same time a gritty determination to carry on and not give in. These fleeting sensations dissolved quickly but I continued to feel a very strong connection with Anna and kept my contact where it was until I was sure that her body had released me, and the neck had completely unwound itself.

I moved my hands to her lower back, specifically the lumbar-sacral area, which felt unnaturally tight. This time there wasn't any imagery, just a sense that the area had been solidly held for a long time. I noticed now that my own back felt quite fixed and stiff as well. I softened it and settled into myself again. I stayed with this contact for some time, offering Anna's back the opportunity to take as much space as it needed and permission to let go of years of accumulated tension. The holding initially subsided and then reappeared again, giving me the impression that the experience of release was itself frightening and exposing. I seemed to be connected to a very fine but raw sensitivity without protection or rooting. This made me feel that I wanted to work with strengthening her spine, her back and her standing in the world, and to help her to develop some very tangible boundaries. I was strongly aware of needing to connect all the parts of her body and mind so that she could start to be all one piece. I wanted her to know the strength of her own back and for it to be a very real support for her. In effect I could lend her my back to mirror the sensation of being secure in her body and of coming from a safe space. I realised that helping her to be at home in her body and allowing it to be a resource would be the main plank of our work together, but if change of this nature was to be lasting it needed time to be assimilated at every level – mental, physical and emotional.

I didn't mention the imagery I saw to Anna, because I didn't know if it would be helpful to her. Instead I decided to discuss it with my supervisor. It felt very much like a cliché, but it did accurately sum up my impressions of Anna and our work together. I was gradually becoming aware of differing facets of her personality but the one that had been uppermost today was the lost child. Anna had not been supported at key periods of her life, and I wondered whether battling the elements on her own had started in her childhood – she had described to me that she had virtually brought herself up. The situation had perhaps been compounded when she went through labour and the care of her baby entirely alone. Life is full of repeating patterns, and I could see how this might apply to Anna. With her history she could easily have assumed the victim archetype but so far I didn't think that this was a dominant part of her personality. She seemed instead to be struggling through against all the odds.

I thought that it was most important that Anna had some breathing space so that she could build up her resources and pick up the reins of her life. Rediscovering her joie de vivre could start to give her a life of her own outside the family. Anna's body had a quality of sustained hyper-vigilance that could have come from her early experience. This had probably taken up much of her energy throughout life. As a result, she had little enthusiasm or drive left for any sort of life or goals of her own beyond the day-to-day tasks of looking after a young family. She might, in time, choose to begin the process of coming to terms with her past and her feelings of abandonment, and as it so neatly chimed with my own experience I was only too happy to support her in that journey.

On writing up my notes afterwards I realised that I still hadn't any idea of what I had picked up in the earlier session when I had felt such an emotional charge in her solar plexus. It seemed significant, and I should probably have pursued it further with Anna at the time, but she seemed to have lost track of it by the end of the treatment. I wrote that she was much more trusting and at ease, but at times I felt that she was reverting to a small child wanting to be mothered. Because I had felt my mothering tendencies coming to the fore again today I decided to keep an eye on this in future. I had been particularly touched when she had described her childhood and first pregnancy, and I know this is something I need to revisit in my own therapy.

## Our Story

### LIZ

In Chapter Three we at last begin to get a glimpse into Anna's background. She has kept her story carefully hidden for most of her life, but when Sarah finally takes her case history, it all comes tumbling out, and Anna slowly starts to realise how much of an impact her earlier life has had. The trust that has developed between them means she now feels safe enough to be able to reveal her past to Sarah, something she has rarely done before.

Whilst writing we looked back into our own life histories and at how we had arrived in the present moment. Trust developed to the point where we could share past experiences and even use them, woven in where appropriate, to illustrate the backgrounds of Anna and Sarah. During our discussions and the writing of this book, we came to a new understanding of the old cliché that, although you can never rewrite history, you can nevertheless come to a new relationship with it. Unexpectedly, this has become our journey too, excavating our past histories and noticing how former experiences and traumas continue to resonate in the present. Because of the cyclical nature of life, problems are likely to repeat themselves, but listening to our own stories and then seeing parts of them written on the page has helped us to come to terms with, and understand, painful memories. I once heard that Jung used to tell his dreams to his gardener, not for them to be analysed but so that he could listen to himself telling them. Hearing a story spoken out loud can both bring it to life and change how you see it. Vocalising something can crystallise what up until then has only been a thought, a dream, an idea or a piece of writing.

At the end of this session, Anna realises how helpful it has been to open up to Sarah. Telling her story and having her words and body listened to simultaneously allow her to relate to her past from a new perspective. She experiences, perhaps for the first time, the power of listening and presence. The counselling she had in the past was unsuccessful, but she recognises how different the therapy sessions are with Sarah.

Being listened to and truly heard is an amazing experience. This is what it feels like to me. For a few moments, you really have the floor. What you are saying is the most important thing in the world. The person opposite you is not just waiting for you to finish so that she can jump in with her own opinion, or tell you what to do, but is giving you the space to open your heart. If you are able to do that and are received with equal sincerity, you may feel as if you have spoken your truth for the very first time. It is a sacred space where there is no judgement or pressure.

This chapter explores the past and how it affects us. We ask the question, 'Where have I come from?' And the answer seems to be, 'How far back do we go?' In Craniosacral Therapy we usually look at our clients' histories of physical and emotional traumas.

Because of the profound effect that birth can have, many therapists will also ask about this. Some will go even further back, to the time spent in the womb, to conception and, ultimately, to the period spent in our grandmother's womb as the eggs in our developing mother. Of course there can be no conscious memory of any of these stages, but if we believe that our bodies record everything that has happened to us, these experiences must necessarily be ingrained and may have a part to play in later life. At times they may surface randomly and unexpectedly, and contribute to unexplained patterns of behaviour and choices. As we write, there is currently new research being undertaken on trauma victims and their descendants indicating that life experience does indeed have an impact on the genetic code and on subsequent generations.

In time, Sarah is likely to ask Anna if she knows anything about how she was born and the circumstances surrounding that part of her life. If Anna has any information it will be useful additional material for the case history and could help Sarah to understand better her present situation. The effects of the birth process can be very confusing if you only look at it in isolation. I have seen babies in my clinic who have been born naturally in what would appear to be ideal environments but who are nonetheless very anxious. I have also seen babies who have been pulled out by a ventouse and subjected to other medical interventions, yet are coping extraordinarily well. Of course, these are probably anomalies and finding the opposite would be more likely, but what it does show is that other factors may be at work. The anxious baby may have been born to a stressed mother or to one who had a difficult pregnancy and labour. The ventouse baby might have experienced a wonderful pregnancy and been born to extremely balanced parents who have helped her to overcome her difficult start in life quickly. Any number of reasons or even earlier factors may have played a part. Wherever we choose to begin to look, the experience of life has an immediate impact and, if it is strong enough, stays and becomes embedded in the body, shaping and moulding us.

Fundamental to our understanding of a client is an awareness of where they have come from. How can we hope to grasp what has led to our client's present suffering if we don't have an idea of the problems she has faced and the cast of characters who have surrounded her? Sarah has now heard about the three major men in Anna's life and how each of them has abandoned her in different ways. Her father left, married again and had a new family; her boyfriend, Steve, refused to stand by her when she became pregnant with her first son; and her husband, Nigel, doesn't appear to hear or understand her. So far we don't know too much about Anna's mother, but we get the impression that she has also not given her a great deal of support. Anna reports essentially being left to bring herself up, and the image that Sarah has whilst working is that of a small bird with a broken wing.

In Sarah's story in this chapter, we show her thinking about how information comes to her while she is treating a client, and this opens up an interesting inquiry. What does a Craniosacral Therapist feel as she gives a treatment? I have given workshops in which I ask the question, 'How do you feel?' As there is an enormous difference in how therapists feel or perceive when they 'put hands on', it is useful for us to share our impressions. Some of us are intellectual in our approach and analyse as we go along; others feel purely through their hands and respond reflexively. For many, the perception of touch is like that of a synaesthetic, mixing or combining the senses. Feeling what is going on internally for another person is so influenced by our own experience of being touched that we all do it differently, and information can come via hands, head, heart or a combination of all three.

Sometimes images or thoughts present themselves that seem to have no relevance to the treatment. For instance, I once put my hands on someone's head and felt as if I was holding a nest full of squawking blackbirds. I had no idea what this meant at the time, but discovered subsequently that this client had severe psychiatric problems of which I had no knowledge in that first treatment. While working with another person, I had a vision of a wood full of bluebells. I asked if she knew why I might have seen that particular image, and she didn't know. A few weeks later she phoned me to say that she had just been prescribed a homoeopathic remedy based on bluebell. As I held a different client's head, I laughed because it felt as if she was wearing huge Mickey Mouse ears. I shared this with her, and she said she and her children had been listening to a Mickey Mouse Club album earlier in the day. As in these examples, it is often difficult to know who or what the images relate to or whether they belong to the past, present or future.

What these experiences tell us is also hard to establish. Often they are inexplicable or irrelevant and therefore I am always very careful about what I share at the end of a session. I am frequently unsure if the imagery that I see is helpful, and some clients could find discussions of this kind unwelcome or even offensive. Overall, though, I find the impressions that come to me during my work useful, and quite often they help me to make sense of what may not yet be apparent about a client or that which may still be anchored in her unconscious.

During this third session, Anna experiences relief from an unwinding process in her neck. Sarah believes this to be fascia spontaneously unravelling itself from some tight restrictions and that it may have both a physical and emotional content. Fascia is connective tissue that encloses and supports every single structure of the body, from muscles and organs right down to the outside and inside of each individual cell. It runs like a continuous net throughout the body and maintains shape as well as acting as a messaging system, passing information and sensations from one part to another. Since it is completely interlinked, a restriction in one part of the fascia may be a reflection of something that is happening elsewhere in the body or may in turn affect other areas. Anna's neck may be either a primary or secondary problem, but she feels relief globally. An ancient story from India illustrates how this interconnectedness in the human body reflects that of the universe. The god Indra flings a vast net across the sky, much like a spider's web. At each intersecting point is a jewel. Each jewel, pearl or crystal contains and mirrors every other. If you pull on one part of the net, you affect the whole. If you look into one of the jewels, you will see into all of the others. Each jewel represents an individual, and so we are all connected synchronistically. To extend the metaphor a little further, each jewel represents a human cell or body, intimately related to every other cell or person.

## DAŠKA

During a session I often feel things in my body that mirror what is going on for my client and this can sometimes make it hard to maintain the necessary separation. Someone may come in feeling sad for example and, as it is such a familiar emotion, I can be unsure whether that feeling is hers or mine. It means that there is a more chance of inadvertently fusing with her or colluding with her expectations of a treatment. I try to maintain a double consciousness of what is going on in my body at the same time as being aware of what is going on in my client's. It doesn't really matter how we perceive; we may use our hands, we may tune in to the meridians or the chakras or auras or tea leaves. They are all just mediums to give a focus for the awareness that is at the heart of listening. It will be different for all of us.

The whole subject of how and what practitioners perceive is interesting. We show that Sarah is worried that she doesn't 'know' enough or that she doesn't discern what is going on in the same way as her colleagues. My impressions when I put hands on are probably more informed by my initial training as an Alexander Technique teacher. Unlike Craniosacral Therapy, where listening and receiving are paramount, the Alexander Technique is a teaching method that aims to give instruction into the most efficient way of moving and living in our bodies. We are listening to what is present, but at the same time we are also trying to project an ideal 'manner of use' within our own bodies. Although I have studied anatomy and physiology I still sometimes don't feel that I know enough about the structures beneath my hands. I am aware of where there is a flow or, conversely, where there seems to be holding or tension and I aim to offer an alternative. I try to discover what may be causing it and to explore whether there is a different way, but often I'm unsure. Sometimes the holding that I feel has a reason for being there, and it is not for me to release it at this time. I remember working with a middle-aged woman who had severe pains in her legs. I could see and feel that she was bracing her knees, and if she could learn to stand or walk differently then I was fairly sure that her pains would significantly lessen. As I worked with her I had a very clear insight that she was not yet ready to release. I didn't mention this but after the session I learned that she was supporting her entire family both financially and emotionally. It was not the time to dismantle her support and show her a new way of being in her body.

## LIZ

I do have a pretty good knowledge of anatomy and mostly have a very clear sense of what I am touching, but I am genuinely not sure whether this makes my work more 'valid' than anyone else's. My belief is that we all perceive things differently and for a variety of reasons. We have all had a different life experience, and this has made us into the people we are. Our genetics, our upbringing, our training in one skill or another will colour how we respond as practitioners when we lay our hands on a client. My own earlier training in Osteopathy gave me a very strong background in both anatomy and physiology, and I often have a picture in my head of the structures I am holding, their quality and density. For example, bone will feel different to muscle, and nerves are unlike fluid. However, I don't always pick things up in this way. On some days it is much harder to know what I am feeling; it is all just a mass of swirling movement, trying to organise itself. Occasionally I will hold a person's feet with my eyes closed and see her body laid out in front of me in infrared like an X-ray. I generally just accept what is given to me at that moment, believing that the way we experience things can change from day to day and from client to client. Each client or 'body' that we see brings with it a different flavour, and we can only hope that we can resonate with it and how it needs to be met, finding the suitable frequency for each encounter. As practitioners we are all subject to variations in our inner and outer worlds that affect the way we touch and feel on a daily basis. If you have not studied the body in the same way as I did you may access it very differently, perhaps by noticing energetic phenomena rather than structures. I believe this to be as valid an approach as any other. The body responds to a listening touch rather than a headful of knowledge, although many people worry, like Sarah, that lack of anatomical knowledge might be a handicap. As a teacher and supervisor, I am sometimes asked for my opinion on this. I always tell people to follow their hearts, and if they feel they want to study further for their own sense of self-confidence, that can only be a bonus. Learning to approach the body in a new way can open up different pathways for both practitioner and client.

I have sometimes come across people who have found that gaining extra knowledge has changed their whole practice and made sense of what was confusing them. Conversely, there are those who prefer not to have too much structural knowledge because they feel it acts as an impediment, and I don't have any problem with that point of view either. We all develop our own way of working, and I try to support practitioners in whichever approach they take.

# CHAPTER FOUR

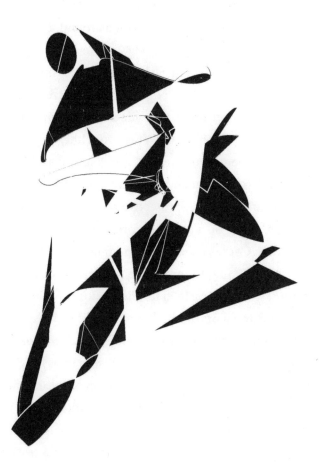

# RESISTANCE

## Anna's Story

On the morning of my next appointment with Sarah, I woke with a depressed, sinking feeling in my stomach and a vague sense of doom. Something told me it was going to be a bad day, and so it was. The children were all in impossible moods. First they wouldn't get up when called, and then they dawdled around, not getting ready for school. Oscar was the worst. He's in the middle of revising for his GCSEs and can't seem to get up the enthusiasm for anything at all, particularly school work. Nigel is getting increasingly annoyed with his lazy, laidback attitude to life and his seeming inability to take responsibility for himself. Whenever either of us tries to pick him up on his behaviour, he just glares and disappears into his room, slamming the door and swearing under his breath. I find this particularly difficult. I feel protective of Oscar and yet don't want Nigel to get upset, so I'm really torn between the two of them. Unfortunately, Oscar's behaviour is rubbing off on the younger two, and they're beginning to reproduce perfectly his facial and verbal expressions, so I think we're in for much more of this in the future.

Partly due to all of this, I felt one of my headaches coming on. This, combined with my earlier low mood, made me long to go back to bed to try to sleep off my negativity. Just as I was heading back up the stairs after the front door had banged on Nigel and the children, I remembered that I had my appointment with Sarah at 11.00.

So far, I have looked forward to my sessions. I like the feeling of complete relaxation that comes at the end of a treatment, and I've enjoyed being with Sarah because, during the time we've spent together, her calmness has rubbed off on me, and I've started to see some light at the end of the tunnel. Today, however, I didn't want to go. There were several reasons for this: first, I wasn't sure that it was working. I hadn't noticed my symptoms changing that much and the calmness and relaxation seemed confined to the time spent in

Sarah's room. As soon as I got back into my everyday life, the effect wore off. Thinking about that made me feel horribly churned up and brought up a lot of disturbing questions. If I wasn't improving was it my fault that nothing much was changing? Was I somehow hampering things, or could I be completely untreatable? When Sarah asked me how I was doing, would she be disappointed in my lack of progress? Would she decide there was no point in carrying on? And what about Sarah herself? Her touch is so imperceptible that I was still not convinced that she was doing anything apart from sending me off to sleep. Was I wasting my money on something that was not going to help at all? Surely after three sessions I should have noticed a difference. Was Sarah a quack, and were any positive feelings I had during the sessions purely down to my imagination? I felt hopelessly confused and guilty.

I thought about cancelling the session and finding an excuse for not carrying on with the therapy but remembered that Sarah had said at the outset that I would have to pay if I didn't give enough notice. Reluctantly, I decided to go for one last time. Whilst on the way there, my perverse thoughts multiplied, and by the time I got to Sarah's I was in a totally foul mood.

Sarah opened the door and welcomed me into the room with a beaming smile, which made me feel even worse. I wondered how she could be so unremittingly friendly and placid. She asked how I had been after the last session, and I said peevishly that I was good afterwards but it never lasted and I had just had the morning from hell and now had a horrible headache. Sensing my unwillingness, Sarah cut her questions short and then asked me to lie down on the couch. As I lay there, the contrast between this serene woman, the tranquil atmosphere in the room and my dark thoughts and anxieties was all too much, and I felt irritation and resentment building up inside me to bursting point. I was so angry with Sarah. Why wasn't she making me feel better? I was more stressed lying there than I had been before my first treatment. Had she done something to me that was making me feel worse? I couldn't relax at all on the couch, but unbelievably Sarah seemed not to notice my agitation and carried on adjusting my body on the table as she always does. This only made me feel more awkward and uneasy, because I was finding her touch irritating today. Eventually I couldn't stop myself from asking why I wasn't getting better, and why I was feeling so stressed. I kept my voice fairly neutral though, both to hide my uncomfortable inner feelings and because I didn't feel brave enough to confront her with everything I had been thinking. Besides that, I really liked Sarah and didn't want to upset her. She answered my question calmly, saying that I was going back into familiar patterns of stress, and that it was because I was beginning to notice the way I reacted that it felt more acute. Even though I was still angry and confused, this made sense, and I wanted to believe her. Despite some lingering inner doubt, I relaxed slightly and decided to give Sarah and the work the benefit of the doubt for the moment. After all, I told myself, she hadn't promised me an instant cure, and if my symptoms had built up over a number of years, I could see that it might take longer than a few weeks to untangle them. Perhaps I was overreacting and being unreasonable.

Although I was now less tense, I was still pretty jumpy. Sarah asked me where in my body I was feeling the most uncomfortable. Because I was feeling agitated all over, it was difficult to answer. I finally managed to pin down the worst place as my stomach. She asked me to put my hand there and to notice how it felt, and put her hand over mine. I was quite gurgly inside at first, possibly because I'd only managed to have a cup of coffee for breakfast. While my hand lay there, I noticed that I couldn't seem to take a deep breath. There was a heavy weight pressing on my stomach, but my hand was only resting on it lightly. I felt panicky and very unsure of what was happening to me.

Suddenly a memory came out of nowhere. Once again, I was six or seven. I was playing with a friend in the garden, and we decided to dress up. I ran upstairs to my mother's bedroom because she kept a dressing-up box full of old clothes there. As I climbed the stairs I heard voices coming from my parents' room. They sounded angry. I could hear my father shouting furiously, and at first my mother answered him in the restrained way I was used to. My parents were very different in character: my father quick and impetuous, my mother distant and cold. I had never heard them arguing like this before; my mother's cool politeness usually allowed her to avoid conflict. His voice became even more frenzied and then, to my alarm, she suddenly began to abandon her self-control. Soon she was screaming back at him, matching his volume and I started to shake violently with the shock of hearing her; it was as if she had become a complete stranger. The argument went on for ages and I crouched by the closed door, unable to move. Suddenly it was flung open, and my father came charging out, and ran down the stairs. Soon afterwards I heard the front door slam and his car leaving. I don't think he noticed me trembling by the door. If he did, he ignored me. I stayed there feeling stunned and petrified. After a while I heard a noise coming from inside the room, and I realised with growing horror that it was my mother crying. I had never heard or seen her in tears before; she didn't normally show her feelings at all. Once when I was younger I had heard my father refer to her as The Ice Queen. I had thought at the time it was rather a glamorous thing to be called because I had just read the fairy story of the Snow Queen. I had not realised then how frustrated he must have felt at her coldness.

The idea of my mother losing control was so frightening that I couldn't move from outside the door for a very long time. I don't really remember what happened next; everything is a bit blurred. I have no memory of moving away from the door or my friend leaving, but things must have somehow returned to normal. I do remember that my father disappeared after that and my mother seemed even more icy and cool for a long time afterwards and hardly spoke to me at all. Then I was told, without explanation, that they were getting divorced and that my father didn't live with us any more. Eventually he married someone else and so did she, but in those few moments everything changed and I never really felt safe or protected again. Even though my mother had always been emotionally distanced, I had found some stability in her impeccably controlled behaviour, but now I couldn't even trust that. If adults could be so vulnerable and so emotionally unstable who would look after me? Something that had been solid crumbled and could never be reconstructed. My father soon had a new family, but I had no place in it. I found my stepmother loud, grating and inhospitable. My father made little effort to help us to make friends. My mother's new husband travelled a lot with his work, and very often she went with him. I became more and more self-reliant as the years went on, and found it increasingly hard to trust anyone but myself. All this came back to me in a flash as I lay there with our hands on my stomach, and the physical and emotional sensations of my six-year-old self were suddenly very real again.

By this time I had forgotten my earlier animosity towards Sarah, and I was very glad she was next to me. She asked how I was, presumably because she had sensed from my body that something was happening. She wanted to know if I was able to carry on, and despite feeling shaky and cold I said I would continue. It was comforting to have her hand over mine, and we stayed there for a while as I told her some of what had happened. It was hard to put into words, though, and I don't know if I properly conveyed it to her because I honestly didn't understand it myself. I had buried this incident very deeply. I was amazed to find myself not just remembering that time outside my parents' room, but almost reliving the whole experience as if I was there all over again. I couldn't believe I was still so much affected by it. My whole childhood was a bit of a mystery because my parents had never discussed it with me. They obviously wanted to erase any reference to their marriage and, unfortunately, I was part of that painful episode.

Sarah asked what I might need to support me both in the present, and as my six-year-old self. This was a possibility and an attitude that I had never considered before. No one had thought to ask me either as a child, or even as an adult, what I needed to make me feel safe. I realised that both then and now I needed the warmth of physical and emotional contact: a hug from my mother, a caring touch from my father. Steve had been hopeless at showing affection, and Nigel wasn't much use either. Feeling rather tearful now, I tried to imagine and feel myself being lovingly held and comforted, and as I did so there was a wonderful melting sensation in my body.

Some time later, Sarah said she was bringing the session to a close. She wanted to have time at the end to discuss what had happened and to make sure I was okay before I left. She explained that traumatic incidents are stored in the body. If the mind is unable or unwilling to process the shock then the whole experience may become 'frozen' into our tissues. We tighten to protect ourselves from the pain, but bodywork can apparently spontaneously 'defrost' those memories. This releasing process may be uncomfortable, but we may at last be able to come to a better relationship with any buried emotions sealed up inside for many years. She added that both physical and psychological symptoms are often the result of holding too much unrecognised baggage in our muscles or other bodily structures.

I found Sarah's explanation helpful and saw that there was probably plenty more to work on, but for now I was too exhausted to talk. I remembered after we had made the next appointment that I had decided earlier not to come again after today. However, this session had changed my mind. For the first time I had felt deeply cherished and I now had a better understanding of my own needs for warmth and contact. This would stay with me for a long while and I now wanted some time and space alone to digest what had happened.

## Sarah's Story

When Anna arrived today, she looked cross and upset. She flung her coat down, threw herself into the chair and refused to make eye contact. I assumed to begin with that her anger was not directed at me personally, but found it disconcerting nonetheless. I asked what was going on and she said she had a tension headache and was even more tired, stressed and run down than usual.

She went on to say that she had had a nightmare morning trying to get everyone off to school on top of an exhausting week. This had caused a bad headache and now she felt completely overwhelmed. I explained that stress and tension can become embedded in our body and that any small incident can trigger a whole cascade of symptoms, usually totally out of proportion with the original cause. This can reactivate stress that has occurred in previous situations, and so it goes on. Something very minor may indeed be the straw that breaks the camel's back.

Once again I suggested that Anna got straight onto the table so that we could work with her immediate physical sensations.

Unfortunately, I found that my own body was echoing Anna's agitation and I had to make an enormous effort to ground myself. Stress and adrenal responses are very catching, and it is sometimes hard to control my own reactions when clients are wound up. What I wanted to do was present a cool, calm presence that would help Anna to slow down, but instead I found myself fighting to get settled.

This is easier for me to do when working than in everyday life, because as a therapist I am consciously trying to be aware of my own responses to what is happening in my client. Today it meant noticing that I was tensing my body in response to Anna, and that both my neck and shoulders had tightened in concert with hers. I felt, too, the beginnings of a familiar constriction in my solar plexus. Luckily, I was gradually able to release my neck and feel my feet on the ground, and by stepping back and giving myself a pause before moving into the treatment, I successfully avoided going into a full-blown stress reaction myself.

Stress manifests in each of us in different ways. It can cause headaches, insomnia, general discomfort, panic attacks and digestive problems, and the variety of symptoms can make it hard both to diagnose and to treat. Looking at individual signs is not usually helpful so I always try to look under the surface to what lies beneath. I began this time by placing my hands on Anna's head. I could instantly feel a furious energy like a wasp in a jam jar. I tried to decipher what was happening underneath the noise by just listening with interest to the activity. The buzziness slowly got less insistent and I was able to leave her head and move around her body. My intention was to give her some space so that she could reconnect with herself. This took much longer than usual and tension came and went in both of us. I noticed again how hard it was not to mirror Anna's agitation and found myself wondering in a moment of doubt if I had anything at all to offer her. My habitual negativity momentarily reared its head, and it was quite an effort to resist it.

I asked Anna to describe what she was experiencing because I thought it might be useful for her to notice how her physical symptoms were mirroring her thoughts and contributing to her emotional state. She unexpectedly burst out that she had been coming to see me for several sessions and that things were no better. In fact they were probably worse. She confessed that she had been thinking of cancelling today and calling the whole thing off. Just before doing so, she had remembered that she would have to pay a cancellation fee so she had decided to come for one last time. As she was speaking, I began to feel the familiar sinking feeling that usually accompanies feelings of insecurity about my work. I so much wanted to make Anna feel better but so far had only succeeded in making her feel worse. I wasn't even sure at that moment whether the feeling in my gut belonged to Anna or to me. Probably a bit of each, I thought.

It was hard to go on with the treatment after this wakeup call. I began to feel quite wobbly about my relationship to Anna. She badly needed me to tell her that she was improving and I found myself wanting to make everything better for her, but I also noticed how much encouragement I needed myself. At that moment I wanted reassurance that the treatment was useful and meaningful, and needed a pat on the head or a motherly hug. I wanted Anna to make it alright for me too, and for a moment our roles were confused. I had to make a huge effort to dismiss these feelings and return to my own centre and a sense of my physical body in space. The agitation in my solar plexus lessened and gradually became one of an overall range of sensations, not the most dominant. My explanation to Anna was that she was probably noticing her stressful reactions more because of the work that we were doing and that this, although uncomfortable, was relatively common. Change requires a period of adjustment and it is pretty normal to feel worse at first. Habitual patterns of stress and tension that have taken so long to build up cannot realistically be expected to change overnight. From my current place of insecurity this all felt a bit thin to me, but she seemed to accept it for the moment, so we carried on.

I asked Anna where she felt most uncomfortable, and after thinking for a moment she put her hand on her stomach. I agreed that this was exactly the spot I had noticed and it seemed a good place to start work. I put one hand under the middle of her back and the other very softly over Anna's hand. All was quiet for a moment or two and I noticed the rising and falling of sensation in her body. I felt she was settling and going deeper into stillness when suddenly there was a jolt that seemed to go right through her, and the texture of both her breathing and her body changed. A minute or so later she said that she could feel crushing sensations in her chest and throat. The agitation in her stomach, which had appeared to be resolving, was back with a vengeance. I made sure she knew I was there beside her, and let her know that she could tell me anything that she wanted to about what she was experiencing.

She eventually said that she had suddenly had a memory of being a small child, which seemed to be connected to the sensation in her stomach. I asked her to tell me, if she could, what had happened and what it was that she was remembering. For a long moment she didn't say anything at all and seemed to be struggling to maintain her composure. She swallowed a few times and turned her head from side to side like someone trying to escape, and her body tensed as if to stop itself from shaking. I was acutely aware of her anxiety and desire to turn away from her physical sensations. It seemed clear that she was remembering or reliving a traumatic event but I had no clue what it was. I'm afraid I immediately leapt to the conclusion that she may have suffered abuse of some kind. Something had obviously caused her system to suffer a huge and unprocessed shock, which had now unexpectedly risen to the surface. Abuse is a common cause of reactions like this, and without any feedback from Anna, I was working in the dark.

When she did begin to speak it was in a very small and childlike voice. It seems that when she was very young she had been innocently playing with a friend and had gone to find something in her mother's bedroom when she had overheard a massive row between her parents, after which her father had left for good. She had watched helplessly and unseen as her mother broke down completely. Anna had been frozen to the spot unable to move. She had felt petrified and completely powerless to do anything. Her mother had apparently always been rather cold and detached and to see her hysterical and out of control had been earth shattering. This terrifying experience coupled with the fact that no one had ever explained to her what had happened or why her father had suddenly disappeared meant that she had deliberately tried to bury the whole event in the frail hope that if she could forget about it then perhaps the pain would go away.

I asked whether it was okay for us to carry on and, after getting her consent, I invited her to think back to that darkened room to see if she could remember how her body had felt. I reassured her that we could stop at any time she wanted, that she would always be in control and that I would not take her further than she wished to go. She replied that it was as if all sense of safety and comfort in her life had disappeared from that moment. She thought she could associate the tightening in her stomach with the time that she was standing there immobile and paralysed not knowing what to do. It was as if she had been punched in the stomach and left feeling winded and nauseous. After that time she felt that could never really relax and play unselfconsciously. She had felt that she needed to keep an eye on things at all times, in case something awful happened again. No wonder her system felt so hyper-vigilant.

Anna had never talked to anyone about what she had seen and heard. She had been frightened that perhaps it had all been her fault. This explained a lot of things. It made sense of my intuitive feeling that we were really working on much earlier issues than those that had so far emerged in her case history.

Once again I asked if she felt strong enough to continue or if she would like me to move my hands. She said that she would like to go on. I was pleased, as I thought it was important for her to begin to unlock some of the emotions and physical holding that had been lodged in her body for so long. I asked her to imagine herself as that young frightened child, to remember how she had felt, and suggested that she might like to ask the child what she needed. Anna was quiet for a time and then answered that she didn't know how to do that.

'Well, if you saw one of your children in the sort of state that you are describing, what would you do?' I asked.

'Oh, that's easy, I'd just pick them up and hold them,' she said.

'Could you perhaps imagine picking up and holding the small child that you once were?'

Once more she was quiet and I was aware of the deepening stillness and silence of the room. I could feel her body slowly releasing. I encouraged this softening further by asking Anna to find a quiet place in her imagination and to sit with the frightened child and soothe her. All the while I kept my contact on her stomach and lower back. My intention was to remind her that I was supporting her in the present moment while maintaining her connection to the earlier emotional memory. Gradually I felt her body responding. I consciously kept the thought of support uppermost in my intention and tried not to lose awareness of spaciousness in my own body and around me. When it felt right to do so I withdrew my hands.

I moved back to her head to see if anything had changed since the start of the session. The nervous quality that I had picked up in the beginning had lessened considerably but I could still feel echoes of it in my hands. I felt tight in my chest and had a lump in my throat and I suspected that Anna was feeling the same. I judged that we had done enough for one session and gradually withdrew my attention and then my hands. I wanted to leave time to assimilate what had happened and so I just allowed a sense of space and peace to develop in the remaining time.

I asked Anna to sit quietly for a moment after we had finished to make sure that she was okay. I explained that our bodies and our musculature can hold memories, particularly if we have deliberately buried them, and suggested that in future sessions we took things slowly to allow her to come to terms with what happened at her own pace. I asked whether she wanted to talk any more but she said that she would rather think about it quietly on her own. She left the room looking very much more positive than she had an hour ago. I was feeling pretty shattered myself, though. It had been a difficult session for me. So many of my own insecurities had come to the surface, and even though Anna seemed to have got over her earlier anger towards me, I was still left with feelings of guilt and blame for her lack of progress. Maybe what had happened during the session had moved things forward, but we wouldn't know until next time, if indeed she arrived at all.

## Our Story
### LIZ AND DAŠKA

It's not unusual for clients to start to begin to feel resentful when they have had several sessions and haven't seen much improvement. It happens all the time. You make a connection over a few sessions and your client has had a positive experience, or at least enough of a glimpse of how things might be different to intrigue and encourage her to continue with the process. Then day-to-day life reasserts itself, nothing appears to have changed and it all seems ridiculously indulgent. Anna is unfamiliar with complementary therapies and the concept that healing often starts slowly and imperceptibly. In some ways this is easier to accept in psychotherapy, where it is acknowledged that things take time to unravel and resolve, but for some reason it is expected that bodywork therapies should work instantly. Sarah could perhaps help Anna to see more vividly that although her more distressing symptoms are unchanged and might even have got worse, some others have disappeared without her noticing. It is encouraging though that Anna is obviously comfortable enough with Sarah to tell her of her disappointment about not getting better. Many people would not be able to be this honest and might just disappear from therapy.

Telling Sarah her history in this chapter unlocks something in Anna that has lain dormant for years and that she has rarely talked about to anyone. Asking the right questions can uncover deeper layers within the client, as we see in our narrative. As we saw in the legend of Perceval and the Fisher King, the importance of asking the right question in the right way is crucial. It is only after a lifetime's search that Perceval is finally able to ask the healing question, 'What ails you?' allowing the Fisher King to heal and the Waste Land to regenerate. Perceval is not required to answer the question; it is only necessary for him to ask it.

As therapists we often find ourselves at a loss when confronted with our client's pain. They may have come to us with puzzling and confusing symptoms, and we can become as lost as they are in a maze of physical and emotional complaints. It can be extremely difficult for either of us to delve under the surface of many years of coping, armouring and outright denial. It is at this point that asking the right question may be the key to moving things forward. In a bodywork context, we may find that asking a client a particular question may provide an opening to a new layer of discovery or a new outlook on an old problem.

So what is this magical question that we can ask our clients to facilitate healing? When and how do we ask it? Unfortunately there is no template; each new circumstance requires a response that arises naturally and without preconception. The 'right' question could come to you whilst the case history is being taken or while your client is lying quietly on the couch. It might emerge as the result of pondering how to say something, or it may randomly pop out of the unconscious. Sometimes you will speak it out loud to the client and sometimes you will ask it silently in your head. What may feel like the right question could lead you down a blind alley, achieving nothing and possibly closing things down. Occasionally, the right question is the wrong question, but asking it may paradoxically provoke an unexpected breakdown of resistance. Perhaps, now and then, the healing question is not a question at all, but merely a passing thought, the shadow of an enquiry. Like opening a window in a stuffy room, it may completely alter the atmosphere.

Trust is vital in all relationships. If our clients feel seen and accepted for whom they are, they can begin to discover what it is that truly ails them. As bodyworkers we try to give our clients a sense of safety in their own bodies and their own skins, possibly for the first time. This is particularly true of clients who have suffered trauma.

Asking the healing question can be the key that opens the door to a new landscape, a new step in the journey. Like Perceval, we are working with few guidelines but if we can allow ourselves to be less self-critical of our own imperfections, most of the time things will go well.

In our story Anna shows clear signs of trauma. Sarah leaps to the conclusion that there may have been a history of abuse, but trauma does not necessarily involve either sexual or physical harm. It is a psychophysical experience and can be present even where there is no physical damage. Any incident that overwhelms us and leaves us unable to process the event and let it go can have the same effect. For Anna, witnessing the row between her parents and her father's departure from the family home is an example of such a trauma. Her description of how she felt at the time is a classic illustration of how we react to such an upheaval on a physical level. Essentially, Anna's system went into shock. She would have been flooded by a massive amount of stress hormones, but because of her overwhelming fear she found herself unable to move. She describes it as being petrified. Whatever the reason, flight, fight or freezing and subsequent dissociation from the body are fairly common responses to being trapped in what we perceive to be an impossible situation. The classic metaphor is that of someone trying to drive with one foot flat down on the accelerator and one foot on the brake. If we are unable to manage or understand either what has happened to us or our responses to the trauma then physical sensations, memories and emotions from that event may all become inextricably locked in our bodies. Evoking one component can also evoke the others. Memories do not just inhabit our minds but can become embedded in our nervous systems, expressing themselves through skin and muscle and ultimately affecting our whole way of moving and being in the world.

Like many of us, Anna chose to escape from an unbearable situation by dissociating from her body and from the whole frightening episode. Inevitably, this discrepancy between her floating mind and the tension held in her body contributed to the anxiety that she was feeling. It also explains why it was so painful for her to come back into the present; before she would be able to release she was being forced to see and experience the tension that she was carrying.

No longer being conscious of a memory doesn't mean that it has gone away. We may have simply buried it and it will now lurk in our unconscious waiting to be triggered. There are echoes here of the Persephone myth and her descent into the underworld. Bodywork such as Craniosacral Therapy is very effective at working with early traumas such as this because it acts in the space between consciousness and unconsciousness. As Anna was very young when this happened we are dealing with more of a feeling state or reaction than a logical, reasoned response. Listening to our bodies and experiencing them as places of safety allows us to separate the sensory impressions from the traumatic memories that have been locked into our tissues. Bodywork can change the ways in which we inhabit ourselves. Although structural changes can and do happen, the essence of this therapy is aimed more towards shifts in mental and emotional responses rather than purely physical adjustments.

Anna is starting to connect feelings and sensations in her body with emotional events in her childhood. As we have said before, very few clients would reach this stage within such a short amount of time. It could take many sessions, and perhaps years, to reach a place where a client is able to relate to her physical sensations in this way. In some cases the therapist will need to work for some time on a very superficial level before a client is ready to connect body and emotions safely. Sometimes even hand contact can be experienced as invasive, and work may have to be done off the body until touch can be introduced. This particularly applies to situations where there has been severe trauma. The client may be totally disconnected from her body and sensation, and very frightened of what may emerge if she does start to feel anything. As with initiating contact, it is always good practice to negotiate carefully the whole process of withdrawing contact. If the therapist abruptly removes her hands and announces that the session is over, the client may feel suddenly abandoned. Breaking contact is, we believe, just as significant as making contact.

The fact that Anna's stress seems worse may actually be a sign that there is something happening; in this kind of work, things often get worse before they get better, and reversal can, perplexingly, be a positive sign of change. Movement in either direction can be indicative of progress. When the body starts to release patterns of tension, there is often an irritation, which can be disheartening because it seems as if all is going backwards. The body heals itself in its own way and does not necessarily follow the client's agenda. Constantine Hering, an early Homeopath, described a law of cure in which symptoms clear from the top of the body to the bottom, from the inside to the outside and from more important organs to lesser. They also disappear in a reverse order to that in which they occurred. If Anna's symptoms follow this pattern, her headaches may well improve before her stomach problems, and she did report after the first session that she hadn't had so many recently.

This is what resistance feels like to us.

## DAŠKA

Years of holding may make releasing more difficult than it needs to be. The fear is that like the opening of Pandora's Box, letting go will free all the evils of the world; we often forget that what remains in the box is Hope. There can be a conviction that it is all or nothing and that to relinquish a long-held grip is akin to opening the floodgates, and the self or the ego will then be washed away by waves of unprocessed emotion. This isn't always the case, but of course this is what it can feel like.

I am very familiar with situations like the one we describe and find that I can empathise with both Anna and Sarah. If a client arrives in a negative frame of mind it is easy to pick up the same emotional tone or flavour and it can then dominate the session. Although I may know that it is not really my stuff, it is difficult not to react when a client is upset and angry and appears to be blaming you for her lack of progress. It is always hard not to respond to these very familiar patterns; I don't know how anyone else feels but I suppose everyone has their own particular triggers. If you have just given up smoking, the habit may be reawakened by someone else lighting up. We're all different, but I have found that my solution is to focus on my body and to notice how I am physically reacting to those habitual negative thoughts. Bodywork has taught me that instead of dwelling on these thoughts I can instead choose to focus on the support of my back and let my shoulders expand; eventually I become less collapsed and I can get more air, I begin to feel different and the moment passes.

I stay with these more positive sensations in myself and emphasise them whilst trying to encourage something similar in my client. All of these reactions, though uncomfortable are familiar and therefore they make me feel safe. It's odd how attached I find myself to my customary ways of being and thinking and, even though this has been the subject of this book, I'm struck again by how intimately connected my thoughts and emotions are to my physical sensations. Sometimes I'm not entirely sure whether it is me or my client who is resisting letting go and we can spend the entire session skating around the edges, not really connecting. It can be an adequate treatment but it feels somehow unsatisfactory and I'm left feeling awkward. If I could have come to a different relationship to my resistance perhaps I might have worked differently and then the whole session could have taken a different turn.

Sometimes I'm very clear that this discomfort is just another story that I choose to believe and that there are many other equally valid ways of seeing things or behaving. I would like to offer a client that same possibility of seeing or feeling differently; I can't and don't want to impose this, I can only reflect that possibility in myself.

## LIZ

I frequently come across resistance to getting better in my clients. Sometimes it's just too hard to let go of old patterns of physical or emotional behaviour. If our well-worn pathways are suddenly no longer so easily navigable we can feel extremely challenged and it may seem safer to stick to the devil we know rather than striking out in a new direction. This is not necessarily what is happening in Anna's case, but there could be an underlying struggle going on that needs to be considered. Her doubts about Sarah's competence and her own suitability for treatment may be masking an unconscious recognition that things are changing. She will have to abandon her current way of being for something unknown. It is an echo of adolescence, where the excitement of growing towards adulthood confronts the need to stay in the secure world of childhood. Resistance is set up and results in behaviour that both parents and child find uncomfortable.

There can also be resistance to improvement where the client feels that there is some benefit to be derived from staying in the same place. I remember a client who had a seriously disabling condition. She was almost bedbound and needed a lot of care. She was really improving after a number of sessions and we had a very good rapport, but as we began to reach a place where she could be much more self-sufficient, she abruptly cancelled her sessions and I never saw her again. I knew that her relationship with her mother had been difficult throughout childhood, and she was receiving a lot of attention from her whilst being ill. I can only conclude that her need to be looked after was hard to abandon and was stronger than her desire to be well. The loss that accompanied a growing ability to come back into the world had persuaded her to retreat back to the safety of her illness.

I sometimes come across resistance in myself so I know what a hold it can have on you and how difficult it is to overcome. It is an obstacle for me too, and sometimes I am at a loss to know how to deal with it. It is like being confined in an airless box that I can't break out of and makes me feel suffocated and constricted. In fact I'm aware of resisting right now as I write this. I feel as if I'm forcing myself to do it, even though I really do love writing at other times. I have no idea at all why I should be resistant on one day and not on others, but sometimes my resistance can be so strong that it comes close to preventing me from doing things, both in my work and socially. For instance, I can occasionally feel reluctant at the very thought of assuming the role of therapist. It is as if it is somehow being imposed upon me and I want to escape to a place where I don't have to be on stage. Once I get going everything is fine, but before I start, I have to battle with an inner voice that tells me not to do it. I'm never sure whether this resistance comes from laziness, shyness or fear of failure. Is it perhaps somewhat akin to stage fright since I seem to fear at times being in front of an audience? I suspect I can easily fall prey to any of these faults or emotions, although on most occasions I am hardworking, reasonably outgoing and confident. So who am I battling with? What part of myself stops me from engaging? Where does my enthusiasm for my work go on some days? Resistance is a tough one to deal with whether acknowledged or unconscious and can take many forms. I personally believe it is most usually based on fear. A fear that may be connected to losing something, of being exposed, of the scary future or of the murky past, but overall a fear that prevents you from moving towards a more healthy situation.

# CHAPTER FIVE

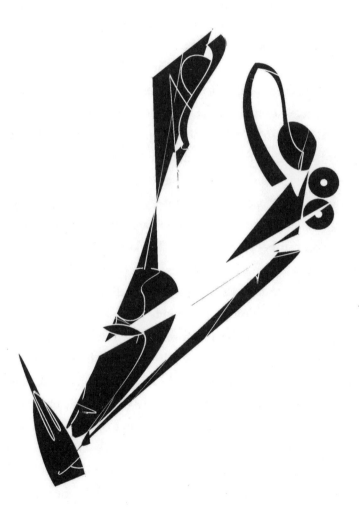

# BOUNDARIES

## Anna's Story

When I went to that last appointment with Sarah I was initially feeling pretty negative and almost ready to throw in the towel. However, what happened during the session gave me new insight into my present situation. By revisiting those deeply buried childhood fears and insecurities, I began to realise how I had tried throughout life to construct safety for myself on shifting sands. My parents were emotionally distant figures, continually wrapped up in their own lives; they had little concept of, or interest in, the needs of a small child. My early relationship with an emotionally frigid mother had left me feeling so alone and insecure that hearing her express her rage and despair was a horribly frightening and alien experience. I suppose this might not seem out of the ordinary if you have grown up in a house where there are constant rows and fights. I think you can become inured to that kind of thing if it happens regularly, but for me it was a new experience, doubly shocking because my mother had a remote and fastidious nature and always avoided conflict. Following this incident she became even more of a stranger than she had been before. I somehow felt I was to blame, but looking back I don't know why I came to that conclusion. Perhaps I saw my mother's attitude as disapproving and assumed that I must have done something wrong. Adding to the trauma of the row itself was the unexplained disappearance of my father, followed by the shock of the divorce and the permanent dislocation of our family. I suppose I tried to shield myself from things that might be hurtful or upsetting by developing a hard shell. It's possible that I too became quite distant and disconnected. I wondered for the first time whether my mother's tendency to retreat was perhaps based on a similar experience.

What ultimately undid me emotionally was falling in love with Steve. The very person I had put complete trust in had let me down when I most needed him, and I was left to carry both his child and the fallout from our relationship without any support. Once again there was no solid ground and I was left floundering. Meeting Nigel some years later was a blessing, but I don't feel that I love him in the way I loved Steve. He is an entirely different character. Steve was vital, charismatic and self-obsessed like my father, but Nigel is much more sensible and down to earth, stolid rather than solid. Sometimes I think he doesn't understand me at all, although I'm eternally grateful for the way he has taken care of me and Oscar.

I was very much looking forward to seeing Sarah again, because the last session had been so amazing. When I arrived, she asked how I'd been, and I told her how much I'd been dwelling on the memories that had been stirred up last time. I felt that things were starting to change, and I was keen to get on the couch and start some more exploring. Sarah, however, sounded a note of caution about moving things along too quickly. She explained that delving into the past like this could be overwhelming if it wasn't properly dealt with as we went along. I thought she must know what she was doing, so I reluctantly agreed to go slowly for the moment. Sarah must have noticed that I was disappointed and continued to make her point by saying that she could empathise with how much of a shock it had been for me, because she had been through something similar herself. I was surprised and intrigued by this, because she had never before talked to me about her personal life. Of course I immediately wanted to know what had happened, and started questioning her, but she suddenly seemed reluctant to expand. I felt a bit rebuffed by this; she had begun to tell me something and had then closed the door and it reminded me of how my mother used to react to my questions. Sarah then changed the subject completely and began to ask me about my earlier childhood: what had my relationship with my parents been like, and did I know any details about my birth?

To be honest, I couldn't answer any of these questions very easily. Most of my childhood is a bit of a blank, and my mother was not the sort of person who would discuss labour or birth with anyone. I was left with a vague sense of unease and queasiness.

When I finally lay down I immediately felt a change. I was beginning to feel differently and was at last able to experience myself in a more tangible way. I was now developing an interest in my body and how it worked. Having always lived in my head I had only been aware of my body when it was painful, and I hadn't looked after it very well as a consequence. Now at last I was starting to feel a little more comfortable in myself.

Sarah described in more detail how and why I might have locked away emotional events in my body and explained how the process of bringing more attention to my physical self could help to free some of the uncomfortable memories it was hoarding. Working in this way shouldn't be uncomfortable, and we were not trying to create a catharsis. The aim was to work slowly and gently to free the body so that the physical and emotional pain held there could be gradually released and reconciled. She asked if I would like to go a little further with what had come up at the last session, and I agreed to do so.

Sarah asked me to lie comfortably and take myself back to the corridor outside my mother's bedroom on the day of the row. She wanted me to remember what it had been like to be there. She reassured me that we could stop at any time and that I could ask for any help I needed. I slowly took myself back in time and immediately felt the effect on my stomach. I had butterflies and an overpowering sense that something dreadful was going to happen. I told Sarah about this; she placed her hands above and below my stomach and reiterated that she was there with me. She asked me to remember how I had felt at the end of the last session when I had said that I had wanted someone to hug me and reassure me that everything was okay. She asked who I would have wanted to comfort me. I thought about it for a minute and realised that I wanted my mother or father to notice me and understand how upset I was. As I became aware of this, I felt myself getting more and more anxious and tensing up all over, especially in the chest and abdomen. Sarah asked me if I could stay with those feelings but also to remember a time when I had been held lovingly by someone. I thought about all the occasions when my children had snuggled up to me, and how Nigel had been such a tower of strength and support. This settled me a little, and I was able to follow Sarah's next suggestion, which was to ask my mother for what I needed at that moment. I found this really difficult. I had never spoken to my mother in that way for fear of being rejected, and I didn't know how to do it. Sarah waited quietly while I thought about all this, but she didn't interfere or lead me at all.

Suddenly, instead of asking my mother for comfort I found myself wondering if it was she who needed reassurance. What would happen if I were brave enough to go and lie beside her on the bed and put my arm around her? When I told Sarah this, she asked if I wanted to try it. The whole situation felt rather silly but I decided to give it a go, even though underneath I was feeling pretty shaky and self-conscious about it all. In my mind, I tentatively opened the door, crossed the room and sat beside my mother on the bed. Uncertainly, I put an arm across her shoulders. She lay very still, but she stopped sobbing for a moment. She turned her head and I found her looking at me with an expression I couldn't read. Then she put her own arm lightly around me. It wasn't a hug, there was no pressure, but there was acknowledgement in the touch. Then she got up, went to the mirror, wiped her eyes and brushed her hair. In my imagination I left the room and went back down to play with my friend.

I told Sarah this when she asked what had happened. She asked how I was now and what was happening in my body. My stomach was much calmer, and I had a feeling that something profound had changed emotionally. I felt almost happy for once. A large weight had dropped away, and in its place was a sense of freedom and lightness. The idea that my mother would need or accept any kind of comfort or loving touch was completely new. Although she was now dead, I was beginning to have a fresh understanding of our relationship. After the session was over, and I was walking back to my car, there were millions of questions crowding my mind. Could I have altered our relationship by treating my mother differently? Had I ever had the power to do that? As a child I couldn't possibly have imagined that I could. Looking back I could see that our family dynamics had been set in stone by the time I was six. I began to wonder how early we would need to go to discover the root of my mother's rejection of both me and my father. Had there been a moment in time that could have changed the course of all our futures and even our natures? I was amazed that this work had prompted my own imagination to create this insight and felt a small sense of wonder that I had accomplished something unexpected once again.

## Sarah's Story

I was fairly discouraged and downcast after my last session with Anna, and meeting my supervisor and listening to her interpretation of what was going on didn't help much. Although I was embarrassed that I had leapt to the wrong conclusion about Anna being abused, she did help me to see the potential pitfalls of making such an assumption. Then she reminded me again how easily I can fall into a mothering role with my clients and wondered if this was happening with Anna. Carol is very perceptive; our sessions are usually helpful.

It is always useful to remember that I have a habit of getting too involved and that I need to be more aware of my boundaries, but I still felt very disheartened. Overall, it wasn't a comfortable hour with Carol because I was feeling so incompetent. Despite her attempts to reassure me I felt rather depressed.

At our last session I had been badly shaken by how aggressive and agitated Anna had been when she arrived. I can understand how frustrating it is if things seem to be getting worse rather than improving, and if clients are used to conventional medicine, they may not realise that with complementary therapies there is often a period of discomfort before things get better. Maybe I should have talked to Anna about this earlier and given her an idea of what to expect.

Later on in that session I had resonated strongly with Anna's reactions to the shock of witnessing her parents arguing when she was young. It made me wonder if I was truly the person to help her deal with this, as I am in the middle of my own family crisis. Like Anna, I was still being plagued by feelings that I had hoped were long since resolved and I dearly wanted to give her the chance to shrug off the armour that she wore as a protection and which I now guessed was preventing her from moving forward. I recognise those disabling constrictions so well. I have learned over the years that struggling and fighting with them cannot correct a tendency to get stuck in habitual patterns of reaction. I believed that the solution was to learn how to step back, observe in the body and then choose how to respond, but that is so much easier to say than to do. I wondered whether this approach might also be helpful to Anna.

When I next saw her I asked how she had been. She replied that our last meeting had been a really important experience for her. She hadn't realised until then the impact that seeing her parents rowing had had on her; when the incident had come back so vividly in our last session she saw that she had never really forgotten it after all and she recognised the enormous emotional charge it still carried. She had been thinking and reflecting all week about the fact that when upset she felt certain bodily sensations, but not knowing their true source, she hadn't made a connection between them and events in her childhood. This had been revelatory for her. She wanted to talk it all through and start to excavate what else might be lurking below the surface. She had been amazed that the gentle work of Craniosacral Therapy could reach such depths of experience.

Anna was excited and was looking forward to beginning the work, but I felt I needed to hold her back since I was fairly sure that we had only just scratched the surface. I didn't want to go delving for other potentially explosive stuff until she had properly resolved and integrated what had come up so far. Neither did I want to discourage her enthusiasm, but I preferred to be more realistic. I knew that this kind of work takes time, but I didn't know how far and to what depth Anna wanted to explore. I have to say that I was also feeling very vulnerable myself that day not only because of my own family dramas, but also because of what had happened in our previous session. Maybe that's why, to my horror, I found myself suddenly telling Anna that I very much understood how she was feeling because I was going through something similar myself. Our work together had reminded me of my unsatisfactory relationship with my own mother. Although she had retreated into severe dementia a couple of years ago, I always felt that things had been left unresolved and that I would never now have the chance to relate to her differently.

I saw Anna's expression change from animation to sympathy, and she immediately started asking some personal questions, which I found hard to deflect. I was inwardly kicking myself as I had stupidly brought the whole thing up. I made an effort to steer the conversation away from myself and back to Anna, but it was very hard now that I had aroused her curiosity. I could see that she was delighted to feel some empathy with me and my problems. This all made me particularly cross, because I had very much wanted to be extra careful about boundaries with Anna. Now I would need to discuss with my supervisor how best to retrieve the situation and was glad that we had another meeting booked for later in the week. In the meantime I thought it might be a good idea to get to know more of Anna's story and in particular her early childhood and birth, but she was a bit vague and didn't seem to want to answer my questions. I was left with the uncomfortable feeling that I had upset her by rejecting her well-meant compassion.

To change the subject, I explained to Anna that tension and stress were affecting her in very particular ways, unique to her and intimately connected to her emotions. Rather than trying to tackle those emotions and buried memories head on, I proposed that we start to look at her physical reactions to see whether she could step back and notice what was going on in her body. It is a very good way of beginning the process of embodiment and of building basic structure and a fundamental sense of safety inside. To compensate for a lack of stability we find ourselves either constricting or tightening to provide an impression of security. I had already noticed that Anna was prone to dissociation, to not being present, to metaphorically turning her back on situations that she didn't want to face. I hoped that becoming more grounded by these methods would give us a good base from which to explore her repressed memories and give them the chance to be assimilated rather than leaving them lurking in her unconscious, ready to be triggered by random events. Without such a strong foundation there was real danger that asking Anna to revisit her trauma could cause further distress.

At that point I asked whether she would like to look again at what had emerged in the previous session and in particular any sensations that she had noticed in her body. She was clearly keen, so I prepared to be receptive to anything that might arise in either of us. I assured her that we would go very slowly and she could stop at any time if she started to feel overwhelmed. Holding the tops of her feet I asked her to imagine herself as a small child outside her parents' room and to notice her surroundings and feelings. At this, I immediately felt Anna's solar plexus contract in a way that I generally associate with fear, and her whole body felt on high alert. I moved my hands to support her there and reminded her again that I was with her and that she was safe in my consulting room. I then asked if she could remember what she had needed most as that frightened child. Anna didn't say anything for a while, but I could see from her face that she was getting increasingly tense and anxious. Eventually she said very faintly that what she had really wanted was a reassuring hug or at the very least some proper acknowledgement from her parents that she was there and very scared. I placed one hand under her stomach to support her and another under her mid-back between the shoulder blades and asked her to observe her sensations rather than tightening up or ignoring them. I suggested that she imagine the sensation of being held by someone who loved her and whom she trusted. Her system responded immediately. She didn't say anything but I was aware of a state of active alertness as if all her senses were finely tuned and she was waiting to see what happened. There was a long silence and a space in which I sat and waited, aware that Anna was struggling against her instinct to fly away and dissociate. I made an extra effort to feel the strength of my own back to reflect a sense of support and reassurance.

I moved to cradle her head and asked Anna what she might have wanted to say to her mother and gave her time to consider.

This time she was quiet for so long that I thought I might have gone too far. Now I had to struggle against my own self-doubt because I remember what it is like as a child to know too much of adult misery and to feel swamped with fear at the enormity of that knowledge. I was beginning now to feel like a fraudulent practitioner as I hadn't yet resolved these issues for myself. Still struggling with my own insecurity, I was astounded when Anna suddenly announced that instead of being comforted herself she had unexpectedly found herself wanting to console her mother. I would never have thought either of suggesting this to her or of doing it for myself and I was aware of my body responding positively to what she had said. After all my years of therapy, it was ironic that it was one of my clients who had allowed me to approach my own story so very differently.

For a long time there was a profound quiet in the room and I consciously focussed on evoking support for both of us. I asked Anna to notice what was happening in her body. I was sure that something had shifted, since between my hands there was an ease and a lightness where before it had all been a swirling mass of anxiety. My own uncertainty began to recede, because I realised that something magical had happened that morning. Anna had found her own way through the situation, and my agonising about my own ineptitude had been unnecessary, although I also wondered if it had been fortuitous. Perhaps by taking my attention away from her and focussing on myself at a crucial moment I had given her the space to find her own pathway. I would need to examine with my supervisor how much my own agenda for Anna might be getting in the way of the treatment process. I was also left with a question mark about my relationship to my mother. How would she have responded to my touch if I offered it to her as Anna had imagined doing? The session had left me with much to think about.

## Our Story

### LIZ

Breaking boundaries can sometimes happen innocently and can be, as in this case, just a momentary slip. For Anna and Sarah there may be only a little future discomfort, but in some cases things can be more serious. Working with couples or people in the same family can be a particularly treacherous area. Discussing one family member with another can lead to all sorts of pitfalls, but is easily done. For example many people feel that, out of a sense of wanting to help, they have the right to know what went on in the session. They may be looking to you to change the behaviour of their family member or alleviate a condition that they are worried about. Sometimes it is hard to resist their well-meant questioning and not fall into the trap of confiding in them. Of course we could always choose not to treat people who are closely related, but sometimes there is a value to working with families, especially in the case of babies and children, where it may be very useful to observe the dynamics of the family unit as a whole. I remember many instances in which either the father or grandmother were also in the room with the baby I was treating and it was interesting to see the pressures being placed on both mother and baby and the reactions they engendered. However, in these situations, as in all others, keeping boundaries as watertight as possible is vital because of the risks involved in inappropriately revealing either your own or your client's personal information and the resulting breakdown in trust. I can certainly remember moments when, like Sarah, I have regretted a lapse and found it difficult to forgive myself. Sarah says she will talk this over with her supervisor, and it is hoped this will help her to see it in proportion. Luckily, the session ends on a positive note, which should also revive her confidence.

## DAŠKA

Because we wanted to explore the idea of boundaries and what can happen when things go wrong, we have consciously invented a large overlap in Anna and Sarah's backgrounds. There is also a similarity to my own story. My early experience was a factor in my decision to become a therapist of some sort. I was profoundly affected by the Alexander Technique, as it provided me with a structure that had been lacking and, like a lot of late converts, I have become somewhat evangelical about the work. If you lack any concept of strong boundaries in yourself, it can be life changing to find them within. I had been lucky enough to encounter a particularly charismatic teacher at exactly the right time, and she helped me unlock doors that I didn't even know existed.

Many therapists, either consciously or unconsciously, personify the archetype of the Wounded Healer, able to cure all except themselves. Embodied in the myth of Chiron, and formulated by Jung, this archetype is common to many cultures. The future Shaman is frequently revealed to his tribe or family by experiencing his own healing crisis and, in the Bible, there is the injunction to the Physician to 'heal thyself'. Chiron was a centaur, a mythical creature, half man and half horse. As the son of the god Chronos he was immortal. Abandoned by his horrified mother at birth he was raised by Apollo, god of light and the sun, truth, prophecy, healing, music and poetry. Apollo represents the principle of rational or masculine consciousness. Chiron became famous for his wisdom and was known as a prophet, teacher and musician. In turn he taught and fostered many Greek heroes, among them, Achilles, Heracles, Jason and Perseus. In the myth he was wounded by a poisoned arrow belonging to his pupil Heracles in a random accident and it was his search for relief from this incurable wound that resulted in his knowledge of healing. He subsequently taught Asclepius, the future god of medicine. Unable to cure himself from his relentless pain he decided to relinquish his immortality and chose death rather than eternal suffering.

Many themes in this story resonate with those of us involved in the healing or therapeutic arts. A lot of people in the healing professions, whether orthodox or alternative, are very wounded themselves. Healing their own wounds through healing others may be their underlying, although in some cases unrecognised, reason for taking up a career in these fields. Chiron symbolises on many levels the perpetual battle of dualism we all face and the fact that resolution can only be achieved by a reconciliation of opposites, a dynamic tension that is neither one nor the other. As half man and half beast, Chiron symbolises this balance within himself. His upbringing by Apollo reflects the timeless conflict between civilisation and instinct, mind and body, and Classicism and Romanticism. The wound suffered by Chiron was essentially random and meaningless. As such it could be described as an existential wound, or even as another example of 'Original Sin'. The story suggests to me that it is our search for meaning and our own personal healing in a meaningless world that brings us gifts. As therapists we may often be able to help others but feel powerless to help ourselves. We are listening to our clients' stories, but often fail to listen to our own. What are our own wounds and how might they become gifts? Alternatively, how might they become unbearable? Like Chiron's myth, our task is to live with both possibilities within ourselves. What may need to be accepted and what sacrificed? In life we often revisit the same hard places and reactivate wounds that continue to resonate for us. Given time they may no longer have the same compelling power, but the effects remain, and like scar tissue they remind us of old injuries. The archetype of Wounded Healer contains within it the triad of the Healer, the Victim and the

Persecutor or 'Shadow'. All three are interlinked and each must play its part. In our story it might be useful for both Anna and Sarah to consider what is uppermost, what is in shadow and what might be holding the balance. To 'know thyself' has always been part of the healing journey; the phrase is inscribed in the forecourt of the ancient site of the Oracle at Delphi.

In my own practice I can find myself torn between wanting to push on through resistance or holding myself and the process back. I have a client who has a long history of physical, emotional and mental abuse. Although he has very different life circumstances, I find myself resonating with his inbuilt reactions and behaviour, and even his language. I have made the same choices, and in an echo of the Chiron story, I grapple with many of his problems on a different scale. My therapist says the very same things to me as I say to him. It is a very strange situation. I have been working on these things in various ways for about 20 years and I still am. The only thing that I can do to is to try to find refuge and safety in embodiment. I am slowly learning that it doesn't matter if I don't have the ultimate solution, I simply do the best that I can right now.

### LIZ AND DAŠKA

The need or compulsion to heal others can mean that we are looking for results and that our objectivity can be compromised. Giving someone enough space to contact her own healing ability is difficult if we are operating from a place of performance anxiety or ego-driven need to succeed. Each person heals differently and in her own time. Meeting someone else's agenda sets up a situation where true healing may be exchanged for a suppression rather like that which occurs with medication, since both client and practitioner are trying to please the other, and the inner voices are not being heard.

It is only by acknowledging our wounds that we can begin to move to a position where we are not unconsciously reacting to their legacies. Going back to our story, Anna is on the verge of an important discovery. To realise suddenly that one has the power to change a previously intractable situation can be an exhilarating thought, particularly for someone who has always felt helpless. Even if recognition comes in hindsight, it can still introduce a new reading of the dynamics of a situation, a new relationship with the past. Sarah suggests that Anna go slowly with the work. Like many clients, Anna is entering a stage of excitement and enthusiasm for the process that might lead to her becoming overwhelmed. The fact that she has hidden these memories so deeply means that she will need time to come to terms with what they mean and further time to understand why she has buried them. We can't change the past but we can, through conscious awareness, start to come to terms with it and begin to recognise its impact on our life.

What happens when we work with people whose stories trigger our own? When we encounter a client who really touches us it can be so difficult to sit back without offering advice or opinions. There are many clients who come with stories like your own and many others who have found similar solutions or strategies to cope with difficult situations but who have come from completely different starting points. In both cases there may be times when it is hard to distinguish what is yours from what is theirs and to recognise that your solutions might not be appropriate for them. It can get very confusing. It's natural to want to help those on the same journey, but yours is not the only path, and there is no finite answer to every problem. As any parent knows, a child does not learn how to cross the road if someone is holding her hand, she just allows that person to take responsibility. In our work as therapists it is our job to help our clients take responsibility for themselves, and how many of us are ready to do that either for ourselves or our clients? Things are never black or white; while one part of a person may want to forge forward, another might be very happy for someone else to hold her hand and guide her across the road. Our task is just to hold all those possibilities in our awareness, without the intention or desire to push our client in any particular direction. We use our hands like this too, without intention but aiming to hold the opposites in balanced tension. It is difficult to put the experience into words because it is a sensory phenomenon. It can be like holding a piece of elastic at exactly the right tension or being aware of acute pain and discomfort at the same time as holding in awareness a sense of the life of the body as a whole.

The therapeutic relationship differs from others in that we are professionally engaged to listen and receive. By revealing her own difficulties in the session Sarah comes close to breaking boundaries. She is actually making things more difficult for herself as she is potentially setting up the basis for a different type of relationship. Sarah's slip doesn't appear to be catastrophic but her habit of self-criticism leads her to magnify the incident and blow it out of proportion. As clients we don't want to know about or discuss our doctor's or therapist's problems; we need their undivided attention while we attempt to unravel our own. On the other hand, we need to remember that the very problems and battles Sarah has had with the legacies of her own past have made her a very sensitive practitioner and may be why Anna has been led to her as a client. If she is able to tread a fine line, her experience could be vital to the outcome for them both.

They are working together very intently on early childhood experiences and Sarah is identifying very closely with her client. Clouding the relationship with her own issues brings a new dynamic to the encounter. If Sarah was coming to us for supervision we might explore with her whether there was a deeper intention on her part of which she was unaware? Did she for example want to be Anna's friend, her rescuer or her mentor? We would ask what practical advice Sarah wanted to offer. Did she want to tell her what to do? It isn't the responsibility of the therapist to problem-solve, and however much we might resonate with our clients and their stories we can never really know what anyone else needs. Ideally, we support them whilst they come to their own solutions. This can become difficult if we have a bias, a belief or a conviction that one way is better than another. Sometimes it's a balancing act, but it goes to the heart of any therapy. Can a therapist be responsive to the messages she is picking up if she isn't open and neutral? If we know what we're going to do, and how we're going to do it before we start, how can we discover anything new? The challenge is to allow our perceptions to be present without the need to act on them.

Anna is left wondering how much of the subsequent relationship with her mother could have been changed if she had acted differently. Was her mother's perceived coldness a projection on Anna's part? Did Anna indeed have the potential to comfort her mother at that time? We will never know. The simple realisation that she could reframe the past was an empowering moment. The downside may be that she might start feeling guilt and ask whether her mother's attitude towards her was her own fault. She has already mentioned feeling as if she was somehow to blame after the row. Sarah might be able to help by explaining that it is not a child's responsibility to comfort a parent. The imagined scenario with her mother may have been the unconscious providing her with a different perspective and encouraging her to come to a new relationship with her past. We never really solve problems once and for all, but endlessly circle our own issues, learning a little bit here and there, we hope.

# CHAPTER SIX

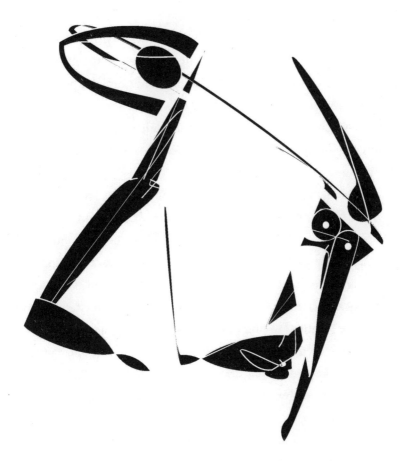

# SEPARATION

## Anna's Story

Before I knew it I was ringing Sarah's doorbell again. On our last few sessions I had managed to get there on time, and I was feeling quite proud of my timekeeping. I didn't want to miss a moment of my time on the couch because I was enjoying it and could see the value of the work we were doing.

In the meantime, things at home had been fairly quiet. Oscar seemed more settled and was revising happily, and the others were picking up on his more relaxed vibes and had calmed down as well. This was a huge relief, and I was able to let go of some of the worries I had been having about them all. I also noticed that, coincidentally or not, my headaches and stomach problems were very much less persistent.

On my way there, I had begun to think about Sarah's life, and how she had tantalisingly mentioned her own problems at the last session. I realised that I had been thinking about her a lot during the week and feeling concerned for her. I had had a long chat with Sasha a few nights before. Now I was making some progress, I wanted to share my experiences with someone who would understand. At the same time I wanted to find out more about what had happened for her. Had her own work with Sarah been so profound? I also wanted to ask if she knew anything about Sarah's personal life. My curiosity had been aroused by Sarah's admission that she was going through some difficulties, and I thought Sasha might know what was going on. She said she didn't. Sarah had not mentioned anything to her, but she had always found that she was very empathic as well and that they had become quite close over the course of her treatments. She still had the odd session from time to time.

When I arrived, Sarah asked me as usual how I was, and what had been going on, so I thought it was the right moment to ask how things were for her too. It was quite obvious from her reply that she didn't want to talk about herself, so I left it at that, although I suppose I did feel a bit rebuffed again and wondered why she had clammed up like that. Maybe she wanted to maintain a distance because it was more professional, but I did wonder why she had opened up to me in the first place if she didn't want to share whatever it was that she had been through. I found myself momentarily withdrawing from her. We talked for a while about my week, the last session and how I had felt about it afterwards. She seemed her usual self and soon it felt as if things were back to normal. I had done quite a bit of thinking and exploring of my feelings over the previous week. It had become increasingly apparent that something had opened up and that I was surprisingly different as a consequence. I have mentioned that a heavy weight seemed to have dropped off me generally, and I had begun to feel really excited about feeling physically lighter as well as having a new sense of mental freedom. I had lost a burden that I wasn't even aware of carrying, and I was hoping that the work today would help me to look further into my early childhood and give me some more useful insights. All in all, I couldn't wait to get on with the therapy.

When I lay down, though, I was surprised once again by the unexpected nature of this treatment. In contrast to the way I had struggled at the beginning, I almost immediately felt at home. My arms and legs felt instantly light and relaxed, and my whole body seemed to be able to drop into the couch and let go in a way that I had previously found difficult. Sarah put a soft, light cover over me, and I felt a bit like a small baby being tucked up in her pram, safe and warm. My thoughts weren't racing around like they usually did, and I found it quite easy to ignore them and just drift a bit. Sarah didn't say very much to me this time, and even when she did, her voice sounded very thin and far away. I was quite happy lying there in my cosy cocoon with no expectations, just my meandering thoughts for company. I realised that I didn't mind what happened this time; I could leave my agenda behind and just go with whatever came along. It was such a relief letting go of all control.

After a while I found myself drifting between waking and sleeping. There were lots of fleeting, random, disconnected thoughts and images flashing through my mind. I tried to catch some, but they were gone before I could grasp them. Oddly, although I felt as if I was dropping off, I was at the same time very much awake and present, and had a heightened awareness of sensation edged with an unusual clarity. It was a bit like watching a turning kaleidoscope that had pictures and feelings instead of beads and in which the colours were super-bright. Gradually I saw that the pictures were snatches of moments of my life, and the emotions that accompanied them, projected onto a screen inside my head. It was the strangest feeling but fascinating and not at all frightening. I was merely an observer with my senses raised to an extraordinary level, watching a lifetime of events flashing before my eyes. I wondered dreamily if I was going to die, but this wasn't as appalling as it sounds, because I felt so safe and comfortable. I imagined this might be how people taking LSD or other hallucinogenic drugs might feel whilst on a trip of some sort. I had never taken psychedelic drugs or anything apart from alcohol, but from what I had heard and read this could be a similar experience. I wanted to see what would happen next.

Although in some ways I wasn't very aware of Sarah at all, paradoxically I was very conscious of her presence and I knew that she moved around as usual, taking up contacts at various places. I couldn't have told you where her hands were though. After what seemed like a very short time, the session was over. By now things had disappointingly started to fade, so I felt comfortable about stopping. I knew that I really wanted to preserve the experience so that I could take it with me and think about it later. When Sarah asked me to tell her what had happened, I didn't feel like talking about it. There seemed something very precious and mystical about what had happened, which I didn't want to dilute by discussing. I hoped she wasn't too upset with me but it felt as if what had happened was very personal for the moment. It would anyway have been hard to explain. Perhaps, too, I was still a little bit sore about her earlier response to my questions about her private life. I asked if we could talk about it next time, put my coat on and left quite quickly, as I was dying to be on my own. Maybe by next week, when I've had a chance to think it through, I'll be happier to share it with her.

## Sarah's Story

I was a bit reticent about our next session, because I was still annoyed with myself for bringing up my own problems. I was also uncomfortable following a recent meeting with my supervisor and was feeling chastised and misunderstood. I feel that Carol has a tendency to wrap everything up too neatly in a way that fits with her own theories. Life is a good deal messier than that as far as I can see but perhaps what I really mean is that my life is much less ordered than hers. Generally, I enjoy hearing her making connections and reflecting on the issues I bring along, and it is usually helpful to see a new perspective, but this time I was irritated by her attitude, and I will mention it at our next supervision session. It is disappointing because what I have gained from the sessions so far has been a growing sense of confidence in the way I am dealing with any problems that I encounter both in my work with Anna and with other clients. Talking things over with Carol allows me to be more accepting of my failings as a therapist, to notice when things don't go according to plan and to move on without tormenting myself. I have a tendency to expect too much of myself and my work and this is not comfortable for me or for any client who has to bear the weight of my expectations.

Anna arrived on time and immediately asked how I was. I gave a very general answer and somewhat awkwardly tried to move the conversation back to her: how had she been and what were her thoughts about the previous session? She said that she had been thinking about it a great deal and was very excited about what had happened. It was obviously all new to her and felt like opening a window into a different world. I asked about her symptoms and she replied that her recurrent headaches and upset stomach were much better although not completely gone. She was feeling much calmer but she attributed this to her life being on a more even keel recently while her son was working for his exams. The younger children were taking their cues from him, so peace seemed to have broken out at Anna's house. I suggested that the relative calm was partially due to her being less stressed and watched her expression while she thought about what I had said. I could see that she was intrigued by the idea that her own mental and emotional state might have a significant bearing on the functioning of her whole family, rather than the other way around. I then asked her to consider the effect that her eldest son had on all of them when he was behaving aggressively, and she immediately got the connection. By emphasising this point, I was trying to help her fully understand that the work we were doing together could influence not just her but also the dynamics of her whole family.

Anna was keen to start so I suggested that she lay down and began the familiar routine of settling her on the table. I asked what was important for her today. Since talking to Carol, I was even more wary of making assumptions about where and how I should be working and had been exploring ways of practising more organically. I asked this question of Anna so that I could be led by what she needed in the moment, and my response could become less automatic. She said that she had been thinking a lot about her relationship with her mother. She had been intrigued by the reframing that had emerged as a result of the last session and she wanted to see what else might happen today. Since last week Anna had come to see the whole incident as a moment in time that had dictated so many of the patterns and themes of her subsequent life. She had been wondering what might have happened if she had behaved differently and what that might mean for her in the present.

Anna's body responded immediately to my touch, and I was expecting to drop into a meditative space. This didn't happen, and I found myself curiously disengaged. As time went on it became increasingly hard to settle. I was vaguely conscious of the familiar tension in Anna's upper back between her shoulder blades, in her lower back at the lumbar-sacral junction and in the stomach area, but my thoughts were disconnected and kept revolving round and round. However much I tried to pay attention, my mind kept wandering. It was one of those frustrating moments where you wonder what on earth you are trying to do, and it all seems pointless and meaningless. I wondered how on earth I could help Anna, and it even crossed my mind at one point that I couldn't accept payment for such a dud treatment. Anna, meanwhile, was very quiet and seemed relatively peaceful despite my distraction. I could hear that her breathing was very calm and deep and wondered if she had gone to sleep. If she had, I could at least stop worrying about her.

The session dragged on, but I still didn't really feel that there was any significant connection between us at all. I moved several times, more to try to calm myself and get comfortable than for any other reason. My skin was prickling with discomfort, and every small noise made me jump. I made a monumental effort to stay with my discomfort rather than to pretend that it wasn't there. Noticing what was happening to me physically was helpful because it took my attention away from my spinning thoughts, and seemed anyway the only thing I could do at the time. It felt better to be doing something even if it was not what I had intended. There are no judgements connected with sensation; you either feel something or you don't. Next I played with the notion of attempting to observe my thoughts and sensations as if they were clouds passing through on a summer's day, whilst trying very hard not to react or hang on to them. It was interesting to observe the connections between my physical sensations and emotions. How did I know that I was feeling bored or awkward or falling into an emotional landscape of pointlessness? At last I gave up trying to either concentrate or divert myself and just spent the rest of the session deciding what to buy for supper.

Eventually the time passed and I brought Anna's attention back to the room. She was silent for some time. I was ready to talk about what had gone wrong and to explain that sometimes a session goes like that; you can never tell. She surprised me by opening her eyes, sitting up and saying, 'Wow'. Yet again I was astounded by an unexpected response from Anna. I asked what she meant, but she was unwilling to give me any details. She just said that it had been a profound experience and that she wanted to think about it and let it settle before talking. I was intrigued and wanted to hear more but I know a treatment can sometimes be like having a particularly intense dream; you need time and space to digest it quietly before you can explain it to someone else. From time to time we all need this privacy, even though the treatment may have felt like an incredibly intimate shared experience.

I didn't push Anna for more details, just smiled and said that it was okay and that she should take her time and didn't need to say anything at all. I felt quite distanced from her as she prepared to leave, but I wished her a quiet afternoon and told her to take it easy in any case. We agreed to meet the following week. Treatment can continue to work long after the session has finished, so I expected to hear that a lot had happened over the following days when she came in again.

When writing up my notes I was reminded of Rollin Becker, the well-known Cranial Osteopath, who often wrote 'S.H.' in his case notes, short for Something Happened. It made me feel better that even he felt like that sometimes, as this was exactly how I experienced today's appointment with Anna! I had no idea what had been going on for her at the time, but at least she had let me know that it had been an important moment. Sometimes I notice bodily changes or movements in clients that seem to be in response to a thought or emotion. Today, though, I didn't notice anything at all and had no clue as to why it had been such an exciting experience for Anna. It's a shame that it was such a struggle for me. If I'd only known how much Anna was getting out of it, I would not have been so concerned about my own performance. Combined with my difficult meeting with my supervisor, I was left with some disgruntled feelings that stayed with me for some time afterwards.

## Our Story

### LIZ

I believe that it is very important, whilst giving a treatment, to allow both yourself and your client a breathing space at regular intervals, so that what is happening in the session can be integrated. I have noticed that the body has an attention span, like the brain, and can only absorb information in small chunks. Consciously moving your attention away, or just allowing things to drift occasionally, can often help to avoid overwhelm. Attention rhythms, as I call them, may happen naturally, not only in a single session, but also over a course of treatments. This sixth session may have been the moment where Anna needed to separate in order to digest the previous work, not only mentally but also physically. Here she goes on a wonderful trip, which she wants to hug to herself and keep safe. This is an example of someone needing time to assimilate all the new information.

## LIZ AND DAŠKA

Like most things, separation is neither good nor bad, but it is a well-known step during the therapeutic journey. The Alchemists describe the phase of 'Separatio' as a necessary stage in the whole process that must come before 'Coniunctio' where Sol is parted from Luna only to be reunited at the end of the process. All elements need to be broken down into their constituent parts and purified before they can be reintegrated and made whole again. The myths of all cultures tell us that we can't have integration before separation. There are many stories involving separation and discrimination. They usually accompany journeys to the underworld or the unconscious leading to eventual rebirth, only for the cycle to repeat. They describe the need to separate from our early experiences and borrowed judgements and discover our own paths. We must separate the wheat from the chaff. The ancient story of Cupid and Psyche has been used as an allegory of separation and growth over the centuries and has many echoes with the myth of Demeter and Persephone.

Psyche, the youngest of three princesses, is so beautiful that mankind begins to worship her instead of the goddess Venus. In her fury Venus sends her son Cupid to take revenge. Accidently he shoots himself with his own arrow and falls in love with Psyche instead. Disregarding his mother's wishes, he marries Psyche but forbids her to look at him or to know that he is the god Cupid. He visits only at night and leaves before daylight asking only for her trust in him. Her sisters persuade her to trick Cupid one night by shining a light on him and he disappears forever saying that love cannot survive suspicion.

Psyche is bereft and, like Demeter, wanders day and night without rest or food searching for her husband. She comes across a temple dedicated to Ceres (the Roman name for the goddess Demeter) covered in sheaves of rotting corn and ears of barley muddled together with healthy seeds, sickles and rakes. Without thinking she stops to separate everything and instil some order among the chaos. Ceres is grateful and takes pity on her but although she cannot mitigate the anger of Venus, she instructs Psyche to surrender to the goddess to try to win her forgiveness. As in so many myths, Venus then orders Psyche to complete various impossible tasks.

The first is again one of separation. She is presented with another huge mound of cereals and beans that she must sort by daybreak. She is despairing but is aided by an army of ants sent by Cupid.

After completing a number of such tasks Cupid pleads her cause to Jupiter who makes her a goddess and appeases Venus.

Here we have the perfect allegory for the subject of this chapter, separation. It is actually one of the few myths in which it is the woman who has tasks to complete and a journey of enlightenment to undertake. The subject of separation is so important in the story that it is repeated twice. Each time, Psyche has to separate one thing from another – to discard the mildewed and mouldy corn from the fresh, to restore orderliness from confusion. For Anna too, things have become muddled and need to be broken down before she can move on and this is happening in her treatment. She is learning discrimination and beginning to discard what is outgrown. She might soon need to disentangle herself and her needs from those of her mother. In time she might be able to relinquish the role of child and step into an adult persona.

Psyche's tasks are accomplished not by direct action during daylight but, in a gentle, roundabout and feminine way, which like so much of our work, bypasses the head. The mind is logical and seductive and you can't confront it on its own ground. Like tackling the Medusa who turns all who approach to stone, you have to deal with it obliquely. Last, and again like Demeter, there is the journey to the underworld or the unconscious. In ancient times Anna's experience may well have been called a descent into the underworld, a journey below the level of conscious thought into a place where the laws of reason hold no authority. Anna sees snapshots of her life during the session. Although the images that come at these times may not appear to make sense, sometimes they can be profoundly meaningful but hard to describe to anyone else.

Bodywork is very rarely linear or straightforward; it has a rhythm and a timing of its own. It is not unlike the experience of motherhood where we provide the support that allows our children to develop and grow, but framework and structure don't have to dictate the direction of growth. It is as necessary to be able to separate from our children as it is from our clients. To paraphrase the trauma specialist Peter Levine, the plaster cast does not heal the broken bone but provides the necessary support for the healing process to occur naturally. So it is with our work. As therapists we operate as midwives. We exist as facilitators to help others across thresholds and to keep things moving so that neither of us remains stuck.

In the story we describe Sarah not being able to make a connection. It's possible that she was picking up some discomfort from Anna of which she was unaware, and this might have been why it felt particularly difficult. Sarah allowed and acknowledged this emotional state and didn't add to the discomfort by tightening her body or rejecting the experience. This ease within herself was mirrored on an unconscious level and left Anna free to pursue her own journey. This could be the root of what happens during weird moments of disconnection and why it is so important to be able just to sit with the awkwardness and anxiety. In therapy jargon, Sarah is 'holding the space' for Anna. Although they are both separate on one level, on another they are very much working together.

Strangely, we do not consider that it is vital to our work that we feel the same things or even know what is going on for our clients. It is enough to trust that although we may not always know what is going on, we can help to bring to the surface whatever needs to be expressed. We cannot always be in the same place; life interferes and comes into the treatment room. Although it can be really disconcerting to discover that each of you has had a completely different experience of the same session, it is not at all uncommon. Often you feel you can't make a connection and yet your client reports an intense and meaningful experience.

### DAŠKA

In writing this book I too have found that I have had to approach things obliquely rather than charging in and attempting to wrestle the words out with the logical part of my mind. It would be fanciful to say that I visited the underworld, but there have been many times when I have had to sit quietly in the dark waiting and trusting in the whole process and it has been quite uncomfortable. It has forced me to look again at familiar patterns of holding and identification and once more try to discard what has been outgrown. I thought I had done this before, in fact I have done this before, but I see that the cycle has come around another time and will no doubt do so yet again. A large part of the writing has been about the cycles of life and I see that I have only been paying lip service to this notion rather than taking on board what it actually means.

Very early in my career as a Craniosacral Therapist I encountered a similar disconnect between me and a colleague in a Continuing Professional Devlopment workshop. This experience gave me the opportunity to explore with her what was going on. Initially I was disturbed, thinking that the fact that I had no idea what was going with her meant that the treatment was an illusion and that we were all just imagining things. What we discovered was that the only important thing, from the point of view of the client, was that the therapist should not try to pretend that something was happening. Sometimes we are uncomfortable or out of sorts and can't make a connection and, however uncomfortable, we need to accept it.

There is an obvious potential for inequality in the therapeutic relationship because, as therapists, we are in a privileged and powerful position, which can be open to abuse. We know much more about our clients than they do about us and our therapy is conducted through touch. We are used to working in this way, but our clients may not be and, as we have said before, the contact can feel deeply intimate. Whilst this is true, on another level however, clients can and do get to know us just as intimately albeit within the confines of the treatment and the therapy room. The relationship can develop on occasion into a surprisingly close and equal encounter.

# CHAPTER SEVEN

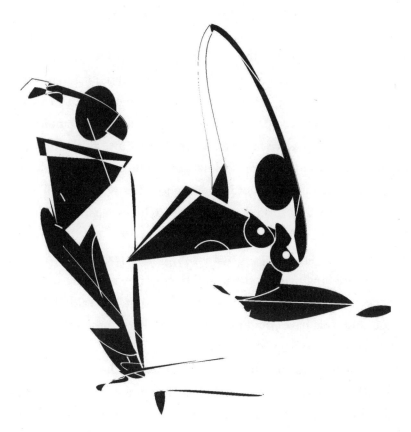

# MEETINGS

## Anna's Story

On the way home after that last session I was feeling pretty spaced out. I couldn't possibly describe what had happened on the table but the effect was pretty dramatic. I was seeing everything in much brighter and more vivid colours. My eyes felt unusually soft, open and relaxed and I noticed that my vision in general was more expansive than usual, almost as if I could see further to the sides and even around the back of my head. I felt euphoric, as if I was floating a couple of inches above the ground. Luckily I wasn't driving, and during the whole journey home on the bus I was in a really unfamiliar space, wondering in a slightly paranoid way whether people were finding me strange because of the odd way I was looking at them. The feeling was still there when I got home, and when the children got in from school I caught them all eying me curiously as I drifted around the kitchen preparing their tea. They looked as if they wanted to ask a question, but didn't know quite what to say. I suppose that seeing me so relaxed and easy going was something new for them, and they were wondering what had happened. In the end, Oscar made a joke of it, and said, 'Who are you, and what have you done with my mother?', but I just smiled at him and carried on peeling the potatoes.

I hadn't told the children anything about having treatments with Sarah, and it was a bit difficult to know how to start. How could I explain that lying on a couch in a room with somebody's hands holding your head had made me feel so different? They would probably find it really funny and improbable, and find ways of teasing me. It was best to keep it to myself. When Nigel came in later, he asked me how my day had been, and when I said 'really interesting', he looked at me quizzically, but didn't pursue it. I had told him that I was seeing someone Sash had recommended for some bodywork sessions, but that was all, so he didn't know much more than the children. I decided to try to tell him a little bit about my session, but I could see him instantly glaze over as he does when he finds something rather tedious, so I stopped and shut up. As I did so, an achingly familiar feeling washed over me. I felt like a child who feels she is boring the grown-ups with silly talk and sees them exchanging patronising smiles over her head. In order to stop myself losing my new sense of calm and well-being, I went to bed, slept amazingly well and felt generally refreshed and better the next day.

Even though the good feelings from the last session had almost dissipated, by the time I got to Sarah's the following week, I was raring to go with the session. I really wanted to get that great feeling back again as soon as possible. However, before I was invited to lie down, Sarah said that as we had now had six sessions we should review together how things were going. She wanted to know about the symptoms that I had brought on the first day. I was sleeping better, my stomach problems were improving and I felt generally more able to cope. My anxiety that nothing was changing a couple of weeks ago now seemed premature. It was helpful to review and recognise the changes.

When I got on the couch and Sarah had settled me down, I shut my eyes in anticipation and waited for the trip to start. Instead, I found myself unwillingly drawn back to my conversation with Nigel on the evening after my last treatment and the childish feelings that had been reawakened. His attitude had really hurt me. Suddenly it felt so unjust and so painful that I could feel tears come. Sarah noticed that they were running down my cheeks and into my ears and wondered if I needed a tissue. The gentle kindness in her voice made me cry even harder. She asked very quietly what I was noticing in my body and whether there were any words that fitted what I was feeling. The only thing I could think of was, 'It's not fair! Nothing is fair!' but at first I didn't want to say that because it made me sound so childish. Sarah moved one hand under my upper back between my shoulder blades and the other below my pelvis. This felt very comforting, and I was eventually able to tell her what I had been feeling and to say the words out loud. By now the unfairness seemed to have got mixed up with some frustration about not having the session I had been expecting. I realised how extraordinarily pissed off I was at being eternally emotionally short-changed in my relationships. This conviction had been around for my whole life, and I just wanted it to stop. The previous session had been unexpectedly freeing and I had been so excited to see and experience the world so differently and was still surprised at how far this work could take me. At last I had made some progress in dealing with both my emotional and physical symptoms and was beginning to recognise how linked they were. Suddenly here they all were again; the conversation with Nigel had triggered all these old feelings and now they were more painful than ever. What I had tried to bury for so long was this sense of being a mere child who had nothing useful to say or contribute and who was powerless and disregarded by the adults. I recognised just how much Nigel had upset me by being so dismissive of my experience, but I began to feel angry with Sarah as well. I thought illogically and momentarily that she was responsible for stirring things up further by getting me to voice my frustration, and this was spoiling the treatment. Disappointment, anger and shame all hit me together and I began to cry harder until I became quite overwhelmed. Sarah didn't try to make things feel better by fussing around me, she just kept her hands where they were and remained very quiet and still. After a while I began to feel a tiny bit calmer. Gradually the waves of feeling that had been so uncomfortable began to recede, and we stayed there until the session came to an end. When I felt ready to get off the couch, she asked me to sit in the chair again so that we could talk about what had just happened.

It took me a few moments to get myself together after all that crying, and I sat there wondering what my face looked like. I am not an elegant weeper: my eyes swell up like balloons and my nose doesn't stop running for ages afterwards, so at first I wasn't too comfortable with Sarah looking at me. She must have realised this as she didn't make much eye contact in the beginning. We began to talk about my conversation with Nigel. I told her that at the time I had dismissed it but it was only when we started working that I had recognised how hurt I had been by his attitude. Her explanation was that when we are accustomed to feeling a particular way from childhood, it is very easy for those emotions to be triggered again. If, like me, you had a family who were distant and unavailable, then every time someone behaves in the same way those same feelings and responses can be resurrected. We become steadily conditioned to respond in a particular way. Sarah said that for some people, early experiences make them consciously determined to live their lives differently, whilst others find themselves replicating their family history over and over again in every situation. They might be drawn to those people who replay roles that they had encountered previously. I began to think about the major relationships with men in my life, and I remembered how much Steve was like my father: he was fun loving, extrovert and completely narcissistic. Nigel is different. He is a kind and thoughtful man in many ways, but he treats me like a little girl who is hopeless at running her own life. He has a tendency to be rather condescending and fairly controlling and often disappears into his own world. When this happens I don't feel heard by him, and my frustration rises to the surface. I suppose Nigel, Steve and my father are what could be described as absent, although in Nigel's case that is not the whole story. I began to worry that I might have been spending my life going round in huge circles and this made me feel like crying again. This time Sarah looked me in the eye quite firmly and told me that life is a cyclical experience, but the trick is to be prepared to meet each turn of the circle head on rather than getting caught up in another round. If you realise what your triggers are, it is hoped you can choose whether you are ambushed by them or not. Once you start to behave and respond differently, others are also forced to take a different approach. By going off to bed instead of staying to have a row with Nigel, as I would normally have done, I had already begun to change the pattern of our relationship. Hence, perhaps, the very good night's sleep. She went on to say that it was possible that the incident had appeared in the session today so that I could experience it again in a safe environment where it could be aired and processed. The treatment that had seemed so disappointing, I could now see as a gift. I was slowly starting to understand how the experiences of my younger self have made me what I am today. Sarah said that this often happened with Craniosacral Therapy; you sometimes get what you need in a surprising way. Before I left we agreed to another three sessions, which would take us up to Christmas.

I went home with plenty to think about. I was not in that dreamy, spaced-out place that I had been hoping for, but I had more of a sense of solidity and groundedness than usual, which felt new but equally satisfying.

## Sarah's Story

I was happy that I had brought up my discomfort with Carol at our supervision session because it cleared the air and allowed me to let go of some of my insecurity. This was good, as I wanted to explore the disconnect that had occurred between Anna and me in our last treatment. I had been reminded again of my tendencies to want to rescue my clients and to assume that things are my fault when in fact they may not be. I was wondering if Anna had felt the same sense of distance between us as I had. The parallels between my own uncertainty and Anna's assumption of responsibility for the break-up of her parents' marriage hadn't escaped me and I found myself wondering again how I could possibly help her. This time thank goodness I didn't engage with or indulge that thought, I just let it drift away. I noticed, however, that I was very concerned with being even more attentive than usual. The previous session had obviously been very important for Anna and if possible I wanted to allow the work to go deeper.

She arrived in a bouncy mood and was looking forward to starting work, but first I wanted to review her symptoms. Overall they seemed to be improving, but I was very much aware that we might be going through a 'honeymoon' period, where a client appears to progress rapidly because of the novelty of new insights and ideas. Any lasting or long-term progress needs to be firmly embodied, and most things take longer than expected to deal with. Change needs to be consolidated and not merely superficial. While your eyes may be set on the horizon, any steps forward are often small compared with the distance you have to travel. The ground already covered can look insignificant and yet, like steering an ocean liner, minute changes in direction have a big effect over time. Bodywork tends to enhance the experience of physicality. Without a basic knowledge of our own external boundaries, we cannot have a real and solid concept of ourselves. Where our skin meets the outside world is the archetypal ultimate boundary. This is who we are and ultimately how we experience who we are.

Anna reported that her whole family seemed to have noticed the change in her and that her household had continued to be peaceful over the past week. Even Nigel had remarked that whatever she was doing seemed to be working. In the past she would have found that remark as patronising as I did, but she had just let it go. She tried to tell him about the sessions with me but it was clear that he hadn't wanted to listen. Although she was annoyed at not being able to share her experience she hadn't let it upset her and they had not had their usual argument.

We started work and I took up a position at her head. I immediately noticed that her system had a softer and more open quality, and the nervous energy that had previously been so dominant was no longer such a feature. After a while I made contact with a quality of profound vulnerability, which appeared to be emerging from a deeper place in Anna than we had reached before. It was as if I was holding a small child; even her head felt tiny between my hands. I sensed sadness and a need for comfort and saw a tear run down her cheek. I asked what was going on and if she wanted to share anything with me. This prompted more tears, so I asked if there were any words or images that were going through her head that accompanied what she was feeling in her body. After a few moments she finally burst out, 'It's not fair!' and as she did so, I felt her whole abdomen tighten. At the same time I felt a pain in myself, between the shoulder blades in the place that I think of as my heart centre. I placed my hands under her sacrum and between her shoulder blades and wordlessly offered holding and support as you might to a child.

I wanted to talk about what she was experiencing, but didn't want to rush her. Anna was quiet for a moment or two and then said that these feelings were familiar, she had been wrestling with them for years, but wherever she turned she didn't seem able to escape from them. She had begun to hope that our sessions might bury them once and for all, but was disappointed today to find herself back in these same old revolving negative thought patterns. She felt that nothing had really changed, that it might never do so and that she was destined to be forever fighting the same demons. Having experienced that brief, tantalising glimpse into another more exciting world of new possibilities and wider horizons, it seemed desperately cruel to her that what had appeared so magical had now turned out to have made no difference after all. I understood how demoralising this could be, but knew Anna would have to come to terms with the hard fact that that we don't really rid ourselves completely of our anxieties. What we can do is reach a different relationship with them and subsequently become more adept at handling them. I kept this to myself for the moment and just listened to Anna in silence.

By now she was really sobbing hard, but she managed to get out that no one had ever listened to her and she had felt unheard and unseen all of her life. For the first time she had experienced being truly heard in our sessions but was now furious that the same things seemed to be happening all over again. I got the impression that she was blaming me for that, and I had to bite my tongue to prevent myself from telling my own story. The reappearance of old wounds is all too familiar, and I'm not sure I've fully resolved much at all. Over time things have got easier, but whether it's to do with the work that I've done on myself or simply getting older, I honestly don't know. I have often wondered if it was not a particular therapy that helped me most, but just meeting the right person at the right time; as I say, I don't know. As far as I can see, the real work lies not in burying awkward and painful emotions, but in bringing them into the light and looking at them afresh. The key for me had been bodywork, such as Alexander Technique and Craniosacral Therapy. I had been so completely identified with the story in my head that it was enlightening to see the world from a different perspective.

Words are not the language of the body and it was refreshing to notice my physical sensations, rather than wrestling with those endlessly repetitive thoughts. I found my experience was so inspiring that I wanted to share it. It was why I became a bodywork therapist. I once found myself during a Craniosacral session, turning towards a very old and painful wound rather than running away as I had been doing for years; it was an extraordinarily clarifying and completely unexpected moment.

I desperately wanted to reassure Anna by explaining that life is actually mostly cyclical but can often also be pretty random, and problem-solving is never as linear and one-dimensional as we are taught to expect.

Instead I said, 'I am listening now and would like to hear what's not fair and what you are experiencing right now.'

I was shaken by the depth of Anna's feelings and very aware of her anger towards me, but continued to work with one hand under her stomach and the other under her upper back. I imagined sitting and holding one of my own children when they were small, quietly and silently comforting them. After a time Anna stopped crying and said that she felt a little better. She said that she had been devastated by her feelings reappearing so unexpectedly and she thought that it might have had something to do with being upset with Nigel. She recognised that she had been reminded of her childhood and had not fully realised how much the legacies of her early life were still affecting her. I told her that in the short term as she was becoming more aware of the sensations of her body, old wounds might continue to reappear but that I was hoping she would find the resources and strength to stick with our work. Continuing to ignore and bury uncomfortable feelings can force them underground where they have far more power to disrupt our lives simply because they are unconscious.

I think Anna will benefit a lot from becoming more aware of the sensations of her familiar patterns of behaviour. Emotional wounds and chronic stress produce uncomfortable feelings of constriction and blockage in the body and remind us of how upset or hurt we are. Continually pushing away, or trying to contain discomfort, forces us into ever-more confined patterns where body and mind mirror each other. Anna will need grounding and support to continue to explore her feelings. I hope the safety of the treatment room will give her a good start. Helping blocked and restricted areas of the body to release should allow her an ability to process long-held memories whilst being aware of her physical experience. In turn this will allow something new and exciting to emerge organically.

At the end of our session I was much happier than I had been before it began. Although I was aware that Anna had been angry with me, I still felt closer and more connected to her than I had done when she left my room last time. There had been a moment of bonding as I imagined her as one of my children and in need of comfort. She had been soothed by my contact, and I found that I had been consoled as well. Very often I get as much from a treatment as my client, and this was a case in point. My own problems seemed to have dispersed and I felt lighter and more positive. Anna and I had helped each other without a word being spoken, and I marvelled again at how much a simple touch can achieve. I had been worried about wanting to mother my clients and had been through some difficult sessions with Carol about this. Here though I realised that mothering was exactly what Anna had needed at this time. Today I had met her where she most needed it and I felt a huge sense of relief and satisfaction; I knew I had followed my instincts and that today at least they had been correct.

## Our Story

### LIZ AND DAŠKA

In this chapter we see how a therapeutic relationship like the one established between Anna and Sarah might continue to play out in reality. Craniosacral Therapy offers a different perspective on familiar problems precisely because it is non-verbal in character. It is a unique way of communicating and lets Sarah meet Anna's needs in a way that they have never been met before. She is allowed to be who she is and is received with no judgement or comment. It is an essentially female encounter; women come together on common ground and although one may instinctively take the mothering role for that moment, there is an implicit acknowledgement that next week their roles may be reversed. At that precise moment this is all that is required. Advice is not sought or offered, but comfort is provided by the simple fact of being heard. In Sarah and Anna's case it is an intuitive hand contact that gives Anna exactly what she needs at that moment. It is only when the mothering role is automatically assumed and becomes pathological that it can become a problem.

Anna's unresolved issues around abandonment flare up and lead to her breaking down and feeling like a small child. She both wants and needs her pain to be acknowledged before she can accept it and move on and she had been hoping for Sarah to do this. She is, of course, unaware of this but Sarah's wordless intention during the session cuts through all the superficial layers and feeds Anna on a fundamental level. The meeting is symbiotic – Sarah is acknowledging her own wounds and the loss of her mother to dementia as she works with Anna and this is why the treatment is so powerful.

As we were discussing in the last chapter their stories are in fact very different, but their reactions to past histories are similar and Sarah becomes aware of this. They have reached a new threshold in their relationship. At the end of the last treatment, they were worlds apart in both thought and feeling. As far as Anna was concerned, it was an extraordinary adventure into a different reality that she couldn't wait to repeat. She was beginning to believe that this flight into dream and fantasy in which the real, difficult world had been left behind was what Craniosacral Therapy was all about. She thought that a few hours on the table had dissolved most of her difficulties, and she had been looking forward to the escape that she had found in the last session. Her disappointment at having to revisit old feelings of sadness when not being heard or acknowledged is particularly deep and painful, as she had hoped that the feelings had magically disappeared. The words she uses are that 'it's not fair'. Sadly, there is no such thing as a free lunch! Even though she has not expressed this in words, her feelings of injustice are directed at Sarah, the 'Bad Mother', for not hearing her needs.

Sarah's instinctive contact provides Anna with the support that she has been searching for all her life. The empathic touch conveys her support and provides Anna with the opportunity to own her distressing and uncomfortable feelings, to express them safely and to be comforted.

Meeting in this way is something that can't be taught on any training course and it's what elevates our work into an art form distinct from mere physical manipulation. This is about being able to respond intuitively in the moment, from the heart rather than from the head. Sarah steps down from her role as a practitioner and allows her own pain and instincts to guide her. This serendipitous encounter is entirely unexpected and unlooked for and comes from a very different place to the superficial verbal sharing of personal information in Chapter Five. Earlier in our story we discussed how to ask the healing question, 'What ails thee?' Perhaps the healing question is sometimes not a question at all, but a moment when both client and therapist come together in a shared moment of truth.

Abandoning an agenda and responding in the moment to any situation allows a healthy therapeutic relationship to grow and gives the client the space to change at her own pace. It is like the difference between a forced plant and one that finds its own way towards the light. The journey may be tortuous, but making it provides a foundation for further growth. The freedom in Sarah's approach gives Anna an opportunity to ponder her relationships with her family in a new way.

### DAŠKA

This chapter was originally entitled 'Legacies' and, perhaps because we made that an agenda, it has never really worked. At the 11th hour we sat down to rewrite and found that, like Sarah, we had to abandon the original plan and write instead about meetings because this was what we intuitively felt we needed to talk about.

In my own life and practice I recently had a similar experience and yet another uncanny example of life echoing the writing of this book. I have been facing a very difficult family situation and have been extremely upset. My own past has been rearing its head and many very old wounds have risen to the surface demanding to be heard yet again. In the midst of all this I had a session booked in with a longstanding client. I had thought about cancelling the session, as I didn't really think that I could put aside my own feelings to be able to work professionally. In the end I didn't and the session went ahead. I wasn't really focussing on my client because I was continually being hijacked by my own swirling emotions. As I was writing, reading or editing only yesterday, the only thing I managed to do was to concentrate on the sensations in my body and stop trying to change them, so I just allowed the feeling of being punched in the solar plexus, the crushing in the chest and the constriction in my throat to be present. I wasn't able to stop my head from taking over and saying all the things I wanted to say and eventually I had to give up and allow that as well. I remember saying to myself that this sensation is part of life too and that amongst all of these intensely painful feelings raging around my body, I could still feel my feet on the floor and the stability and uprightness of my spine.

At the end of the session, like Anna, my client sat up and said that it had been an extraordinarily profound session for her. She had had an experience of what she described as 'allowance' when she accepted that she wasn't perfect and her experience of her body wasn't constant. She too stopped trying to prevent her thoughts and just accepted herself for what she was at that moment.

How often do meetings like this happen? Sometimes however much you try you don't meet and you misunderstand each other. We describe it as being on a different wavelength. Occasionally though, and often at the most unexpected moments, everything falls into place. It feels like a moment of grace.

# CHAPTER EIGHT

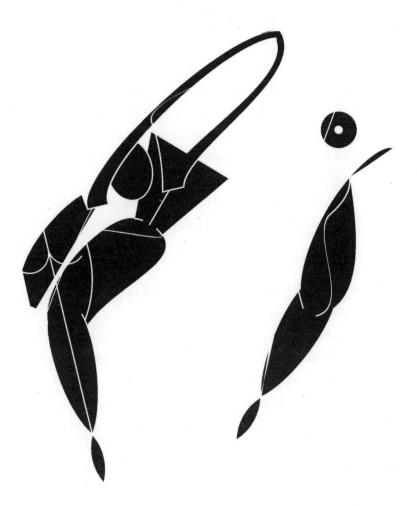

# DESPONDENCY

## Anna's Story

Over the past week I had a lot to think about. The treatment had really brought home to me how deeply hurt I had been, both by my parents and subsequently by my partners. The words 'It's not fair' had welled up out of the very depths of my pain and loss. I had spoken as a child, but the words were those of a woman who was still looking for the acknowledgement that she had been denied throughout life. I desperately wanted someone to hear me and to take notice. I knew now that my voice had never been heard because I had no idea what my own needs were, and I had been ignored and overlooked. I had been shouting soundlessly for all these years, and no one had listened or understood what I had to say.

As the days went on, I found this my playing on my mind more and more. I realised that no one took me seriously and saw that I had become so used to being seen as a coping, unemotional person that I had submerged a lot of my feelings of anger and resentment, particularly towards Nigel. I had come to believe that I had very little hope of being heard if I needed attention. Nigel is not a monster, but we come from similar family backgrounds, where emotion is a dirty word. I was now beginning to realise that I had ended up back in my childhood situation: unable to ask for comfort or attention when I needed it, because I am scared they will be denied. Very often when I have tried to talk to Nigel about things that were troubling me we have ended up in stupid childish arguments, out of extreme frustration on my side and a refusal on his to get involved. His inability to cope when I lose my temper makes him shut me out even further. The last session with Sarah had given me an insight into how I could be more open about my feelings and possibly change and encourage Nigel to respond differently. I had learnt that prejudging situations might dictate their outcome; we can become stuck in a self-perpetuating cycle. If instead of turning a deaf ear I believed that there was even a slight possibility that Nigel would listen, I might be rewarded with his attention. My own past experience was standing in the way of any possible progress. I decided that when he came home, I would try to talk to him. I wanted to share my discoveries and tell him how I thought I was changing and I felt full of hope that I was at last finding a more adult voice.

I thought I had chosen my moment well. We had been laughing about something funny one of the children had said and noticing how fast they were growing up when I turned to Nigel and asked whether he had noticed any changes in me recently. He replied that he thought I had been a bit less stressed than usual. I thought this was a good start, so I said that the work I had been doing with Sarah was really helping and I would like to share with him what had been happening in the sessions. He asked what she did, and I tried to explain that I just lay on the table and Sarah showed me how to be more comfortable in my body. I told him that although she often held my head and might put a hand under my back, she didn't seem to be doing anything at all most of the time. I saw a look of disbelief on his face and then he started to look angry. He interrupted my explanation and became really condescending about the whole thing. He told me in so many words that I was stupid to believe what Sarah was telling me. How could anything so incomprehensible possibly be of any benefit? It sounded really new agey and flaky and if I thought that was a sensible way to spend money, I must be going bonkers.

I completely lost my cool then, all my good intentions went out of the window and I began shouting that he didn't understand or care for me and didn't seem to realise how ill I had been feeling before I went to see Sarah. He gave me a weary look and announced he was off to the pub and that he hoped I'd be in a better mood when he got back. I was completely deflated. All my new resolutions hadn't produced the result I wanted. Perhaps the whole thing was as far-fetched as he clearly believed, and I had only imagined that I was feeling better. I wondered again whether Sarah was hypnotising me into believing that things were changing when they weren't. I had actually just proved that they weren't with my show of childish rage. I decided I would give Nigel the cold shoulder for a while, and by the time he got back from the pub I had gone to bed. My silent treatment lasted a few days. Nigel did not apologise, and neither did I, and I didn't bother to mention that I was going to see Sarah again the following week. All in all it was a difficult time, with Oscar finishing his exams and behaving badly again and the others joining in. My symptoms were increasing once more and it felt as if I was right back at square one. By the time my appointment rolled around, I was really despondent about the whole process.

I walked into Sarah's room feeling awful and explained what had happened during the week. We talked about the row with Nigel, my disappointment that he still doesn't listen to me and his scepticism about the treatments I had been having. She said that often a partner can feel uneasy and left out by changes they see taking place. It can happen with any therapy where emotional holding is released. Nigel might find it uncomfortable to witness me going through something he sees as incomprehensible and worry that I am changing into someone he doesn't recognise. After all, he hasn't signed up for a course of Craniosacral Therapy. His way of handling it is to ridicule it and get angry. Being unused to expressing his own feelings, he might be reluctant to discuss anyone else's. Going to the pub was probably his subconscious way of dealing with the issue and escaping confrontation. While she was talking I began to wonder whether Nigel's own childhood had had an emotional impact on him; like mine it had been fairly bleak. For the first time I began to ask myself if we had similar wounds. This was an intriguing thought.

Was this what had drawn us to each other? Had I been so wrapped up in my own sense of abandonment that I had not recognised it in him too?

Seeing things from this different perspective was an eye opener, and I got on the couch believing that I could perhaps cope with the session today a little better than I had expected. Sarah started asking how I was feeling, and for the first time I really understood what she meant. Slowly I am making more sense of the impressions I get from my body. I noticed immediately that I was really buzzy, my thoughts were racing and overall I felt a bit hot and jangled. At the same time, and in stark contrast, I was aware of a sense of sadness and depression. It was as if I was trying to cope with lots of disconnected things all at the same time. I told Sarah this, and she asked me if there were specific internal places where those different feelings were located. I tried to focus on my impressions a bit more. The jangly, angry feeling seemed to be in my solar plexus. The sadness was harder to place; it was much more global, and I couldn't really track it down to any one spot. Sarah said that she first wanted to work with the sensation of anger and put her hand on my stomach near the centre. She asked if this was the right place, and I nodded, because her touch felt good. She kept her hand exactly where it was, and I gradually found myself getting even more hot and angry. It was as if I was going to blow a fuse, as I had done that evening with Nigel. The heat intensified, but just as I was about to ask her to move her hand away because it was becoming too much, I noticed a loosening. Something tight had let go, and I found myself able to breathe again. I hadn't noticed that I had been holding my breath. I let out a long sigh, my stomach began to feel really soft and rather gurgly and there was a great sense of relief from the tension that I had been holding. As Sarah moved around me to different places, I felt light and almost euphoric. This wasn't the same unearthed lightheadedness of a couple of sessions ago, it was a much deeper and more physical experience. My body felt expansive and open, and I was aware of a new sense of trust. Soon after this the session finished. I asked Sarah for her thoughts on what had happened during the treatment. She said that she had been drawn to working on my liver area after I had told her that my anger might be located in the solar plexus. She had initially felt that it was very tight and hot, but while her hand was resting there something seemed to soften and much of the tightness dissolved. She went on to explain that in her small experience of Chinese medicine an unbalanced liver can either give rise to extreme anger or else an inability to express any anger at all. She thought that I might have stored a lot of my repressed feelings in my liver; apparently this is not uncommon. Liver imbalance could also be characterised as feelings of frustration or inner conflict. Furthermore, she wondered if the stuck unexpressed emotion she had felt might be the cause of my stomach problems and headaches. When the area released, she had felt an increased flow of energy, which would have circulated around the body. What she said made sense on some level since it corresponded with my own feelings of lightness and expansion. The depression and sadness had lifted away as well. I don't know anything about Chinese medicine, but certainly what she said rang true. I wondered how Nigel would react if I told him about my 'stuck' liver and imagined his horrified face, but I decided to be a little kinder to him. I had realised that he may be finding it difficult to cope with his own repressed emotions and experiences far outside his frame of reference. The best I could do to help him would be to carry on with my own therapy and hope that in time he would find his own way through.

## Sarah's Story

I could tell that something was wrong with Anna the moment I opened the door. There was no light in her eyes and she looked completely defeated.

I welcomed her in but before I could ask her how she was, she started to tell me that she was furious with Nigel. She had left feeling quite happy after our last session and this feeling had continued into the evening. She had realised through our work that there were different ways of perceiving and reacting to things, and because she wanted to practise this, she had decided to have another go at interesting Nigel in her discoveries. He had listened for a moment and then interrupted her to give his opinion of what was wrong with her and how he thought she should fix it. He said he couldn't quite see how me putting my hands on Anna could make the slightest difference to her symptoms and it was probably all mumbo jumbo. If she thought it was helping, it was probably just a placebo effect and a complete waste of money. Anna had found his comments and attitude extremely patronising (and I remembered that I had already formed this impression of Nigel myself) but instead of ignoring him this time, she told him flatly that she thought he didn't want to engage with discussing it because it was too far outside his comfort zone. Gradually an argument had developed, which had led to Nigel storming off to the pub and Anna sobbing in her bedroom. I was reminded of the scene she had described between her parents, although at this point I didn't think it would be helpful to bring this to her attention. Since then they had barely spoken, and things were further complicated by the fact that Oscar's exams had finished and he was letting off steam. He was disturbing the younger children by coming in noisily and late, and this didn't help either their routine or her relations with Nigel, so she felt right back where she had started. She had even had a migraine the day before.

I tried to reassure her by explaining once again that it is common for things to go up and down and even to get worse before they get better, and warned that there can be difficulties in trying to talk about change before it has had a chance to really bed in. Here we were looking at a mirror image of the principle that we had talked about at the start of the last session. At that time she had felt calm and peaceful inside and it had radiated out into her dealings with her family. Now she was picking up and reacting to her family's negativity.

It is difficult to describe the physical experience of bodywork to someone who hasn't had it. Although I wanted to advise Anna not to discuss things with Nigel because a lot can get lost in translation, I wanted to be subtle in what I said, as I didn't want to influence her. Anna now understood that her mind and body were connected in a far more intimate way than she had previously imagined. She had believed in the past that doctors dealt with her physical body and that psychotherapists dealt with mental or emotional problems. She had been excited to realise that things could be approached in a far more organic and integrated way. She was beginning to discover the extent to which she was haunted by her past and that she was still reacting from that uncomfortable place. Nigel had not been on this journey with her, so we talked about how she might approach future conversations with him in a way that would allow him to engage on his own terms.

It was time to start working and moving from thought to feeling, so I got Anna on the table and asked her to let me know what she was noticing today. She was considerably more at ease than she had been up to now and able to put her thoughts aside and engage with sensation. I felt through my hands an anxious and restless nervous energy coursing through her system, rather like a caffeine buzz. Underlying this there was flatness and a sense that she was running on empty. Her superficial jitteriness was masking a deeper and more profound need for resourcing and support. I could understand why she and Nigel had clashed; Anna was being pulled in so many directions at the same time. I know when I am feeling overtired or overstimulated, I sometimes find myself picking a quarrel as a way of defusing my discomfort, or rationalising my feelings, and Anna had very likely done the same. What she had really needed from Nigel was some form of comfort and physical reassurance, but because they both find it hard to express themselves emotionally, they had ended up fighting instead. To help her find a way through this, I suggested she tell me again about her encounter with Nigel so that together we could notice what was happening to her viscerally whilst she was talking.

Initially, Anna's whole body seemed to be fighting itself. There was an intensely stuck focus around the right diaphragm, overlaying a frantic surging movement. I had the distinct impression that she was trying to clamp down on her fury and put the brakes on so as not to feel any discomfort, but it was hard work to contain her feelings. I asked her to let me know where she was feeling most discomfort. She vaguely indicated her stomach and I moved there asking her if I was in the right place. After a time I found my hand moving to the right and waited with one hand beneath and one hand on top of her body. I had no particular intention, other than to create a safe and quiet space where anything relevant might surface. My habit of wanting to make everything better needed to be firmly restrained so that this could happen naturally. I do believe that somewhere inside, each person knows what their body needs better than I do. I tried to ignore the inner voices that were telling me to do something more proactive and just sat there and waited. At first our combined attention appeared to make things much worse, and I found it hard not to intervene in some way to relieve Anna's obvious discomfort. After a time I found my upper hand twisting around.

It was almost as if the tension was tangible and I was able to draw it slowly and gently away from her body. I noticed a softening and expansion that spread throughout her whole system and she gave a deep sigh. I listened to what appeared underneath the tension and became aware of an underlying sadness and feeling of hopelessness, of exhaustion at a very deep level. For the rest of the session I was very aware of my own support, the sense of my back and my feet on the ground, whilst working at releasing her shoulders and trying to establish a solid connection between her head and the whole of her back.

When she got off the table Anna said that she felt calmer and more positive. Her face had softened and her shoulders had released, showing that a lot of her nervous tension had dissipated. She wanted to know what I had felt and although I was more interested in her experience of the session, I fed back to her some of my impressions. I said that in Chinese medicine the liver is considered to be the master planner of the body. An imbalance in its energies might result either in feelings of being stuck and unable to express anger or conversely that anger cannot be contained. Traditionally, disruptions to liver energies can be expressed as headaches or an inability to think clearly or to make decisions. It was interesting to me that Anna had arrived for her session angry and confused and with a headache. I was a bit wary of saying this because it sounded too glib and neat, so I explained that I didn't really know much about Chinese medicine beyond what I had just described. I wondered afterwards if I should have mentioned it at all because I didn't want Anna thinking that she had anything seriously physically wrong with her.

Whenever I have been the client myself, I have found it really helpful to hear my therapist's reflections on the session, but sometimes I find it hard to know what to say to a client. My perceptions can be fleeting, impressionistic images that make sense to me but may not to anyone else, and I don't want to impose anything that will worry or confuse them. However, from time to time, when I have fed back something that was incomprehensible to me, it has been helpful to a client either immediately or later.

I want to talk to my supervisor again about what to say to clients in this sort of situation. I think I veer between saying either too much or not enough, and I'm never really sure whether I should share the imagery that I see. I also want to discuss the mechanics of touch and how to touch without intention. I think that Carol consistently feels that she is directly in contact with muscle, bone or fascia, whereas I don't and it worries me. I know that some practitioners always feel tidal pulls and rhythms in the body, and from time to time I do too but not always. I do know, however, where someone is holding tension and usually if that tension has an emotional component. I hope this is enough. I think Anna went home feeling more balanced, and I trust she will have a good week and perhaps make peace with Nigel and her family.

I enjoyed working with Anna today and found the session particularly satisfying. The experience of delicately drawing out the tension that I had felt in Anna's abdomen had a quality of stretching a very fine and fragile membrane and it felt as if a corner had been turned.

## Our Story
### DAŠKA

Anna brings her anger and sadness about her situation and we begin to see an awakening of her felt sense emerging. Having had a taste of another outlook this sense of stagnation is especially bitter. Anna is at last inhabiting herself in a more grounded and connected way than before. She talks about trusting her body, a concept that she may not have recognised in earlier sessions. The treatment is inching forward, even if at times it seems as if it is one step forward and two steps back. Change often happens in very subtle layering, difficult to detect, but very much regulated by the capacity of the client and not by the intention of the therapist. If Anna's change of perspective is going to be anything more than window dressing, Sarah knows it needs time for it to be assimilated. She has a new way of looking at things, a new way of being in her skin. After the first flush of excitement it can be a huge shock to discover how far-reaching the implications of this realisation can be. It is very disheartening to have had the experience of seeing with fresh eyes only to go home and find yourself in the same old patterns as before.

In the Alexander world this despondency is known as 'Alexander's Gloom', the realisation of the distance that we will have to travel and how fundamental that journey will have to be. The goal at this point is to try to find a balance between the excitement of the breakthroughs and the despondency and despair that come with discovering that nothing has really changed at all. It is a very delicate stage in any therapy. We cannot exist in either state for long but so often I find myself falling into the trap of believing each state to be permanent and that I must find my way between these opposing positions.

I have felt Anna's despair many times, when everything feels slightly out of reach and the effort to attempt the task or the goal seems ludicrous and pretentious to even consider. After a taste of another outlook this sense of stagnation can be especially bitter. Physically there is lethargy and an accompanying brain fog that makes even the simplest task seem insurmountable. This condition is difficult to write or talk about with any fluency, as when you are in that state why would you want to write or talk about it? When you aren't, why would you want to revisit it? The worst place to be is the mind with its reasonable and logical pessimism sucking the life out of anything. Far better to be in the body to see if there is a way of being that can preserve the integrity of both viewpoints without landing on either side. In the therapeutic world this is described as 'holding the opposites', neither is exclusively true but both must be honoured.

It is a well-known stage in the great myth of the Hero's Journey. Why should it be any different for us? This stage corresponds to the story of Christian and 'The Slough of Despond' from the Pilgrim's Progress. In the Demeter myth this is the time when the goddess withdraws from the world and refuses to allow growth. In the myth of Perceval we see both the Fisher King and his country wasting away; there is stagnation both within and without. Time has to pass before a new order can be accepted and integrated. I don't think any therapy or medication can help to speed up this phase. It's whatever soothes the way; do you opt for the epidural or do you breathe your way through? It's being stuck in the doldrums; the journey has begun but we still have to plough through the same old ground. I have often described it as being stuck in the supermarket car park of life. We hear about it again in the Iliad when the Greek fleet lies becalmed waiting for the wind that will take them to Troy at the start of the Trojan wars. Agamemnon even sacrifices his eldest daughter, Iphigenia, to appease the gods and the winds do eventually change. Greek myths are rarely what they seem and I suppose that one of the things that we can take from this story is that sometimes we might need to relinquish a long-held and cherished point of view or belief system to allow the space for something new to emerge. Before we are driven to this conclusion we may just need to sit it out. The process is not to be rushed through, but experienced and acknowledged. A therapist should not make light of it or try to make it better.

If Anna were my client I might suggest that she try to notice what these familiar emotions actually feel like in the body; most of the so-called 'negative' emotions involve a tightening of one kind or another and it can be a very simple process of letting them go and allowing the subsequent calm sensations to radiate into the mind. It is often easier than trying to reason with or pacify our thoughts. Another way forward could be to turn towards the negative directly and work though the discomfort in order to discover what might lie beyond.

### LIZ AND DAŠKA

Anna is facing a crisis common to many of us in the middle part of our lives. She has reached a point where her old life choices and ways of being in the world are no longer working; they can't co-exist with a new way of looking at things. The myths tell us that the weary struggle through the troughs are just as much a part of our path as the exhilarating passes through the high mountain peaks with their breathtaking views and treacherous descents. Like any transition, for example adolescence or menopause, the passage is rarely smooth. Clients often arrive in treatment because something needs to change, and they have tried everything else. In Anna's story physical signals are being expressed by her body and she has potentially reached a turning point. She will not be able to get her own needs met in an adult way unless she can identify them, and these first steps into the life of the body are a good way to proceed. We show Anna as a little girl wanting approval from her husband for her achievements and identifying with the position of the 'Victim'. It might be appropriate to suggest that a client like Anna also talks to a professionally trained psychotherapist. Traditional psychotherapy and bodywork function very well together, grounding the experience and preventing it from becoming too intellectual.

We can't change and simultaneously stay the same, and this inevitably extends to our relations with our families and close friends. This is yet another of the messages contained within Demeter's myth. Persephone returns to earth and to her mother Demeter, but she has symbolically eaten the three pomegranate seeds and will return to Hades for the three winter months of the year. Now she has tasted the fruit of the underworld she has been forced to change and she cannot resume the carefree existence that she lived before. She will stop being so dependent on her mother, assuming her own role and passage through life. As Demeter found, it can be hard to let go and to allow change but it is the natural order of things. In our society, time in the underworld is frequently viewed as something to be avoided or medicated; it would be more helpful to respect it as part of the cyclical process of birth, death and renewal. Although sometimes necessary, medication can frequently mask and sanitise the lessons of the encounter and keep us circling around the same issues indefinitely.

Sarah is walking a careful line with Anna and not expecting too much from each session. She is helping her to recognise some of the patterns of change as they shift and settle. As she observes, it is important to move at the client's pace and not to force your own views as a therapist on to someone else. This is particularly relevant here, where Sarah is having a strong negative impression of the unfortunate Nigel. This is the first time that Anna has really experienced the life of her body as an entity in its own right rather than something to be managed or tolerated. It is tempting to try to make everything better so that the treatments are seen to be successful, but this is primarily serving the needs of the therapist rather than those of the client. Sarah doesn't attempt to make Anna feel better by assuming responsibility for her disappointment and anger because things haven't played out as she was hoping.

Providing your client with what she is asking for is a temptation that can be difficult to pass up. There are many ways in which a therapist could work with this but Sarah mirrors to Anna the strength and safety within her own system, which is a sound place to start.

# CHAPTER NINE

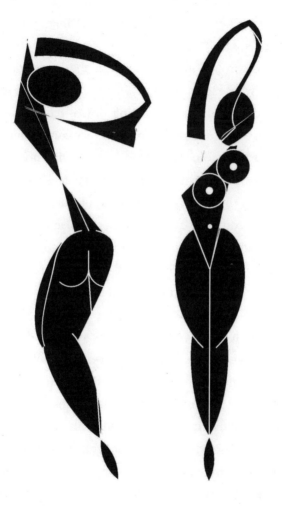

# ACCEPTANCE

## Anna's Story

During the weeks following my eighth session with Sarah I discovered that I was responding to it differently than to earlier treatments. I found that I was neither on cloud nine, in the depths of despondency nor disappointed that nothing was changing. Looking back I saw that I had been seesawing between these differing states throughout the course of the work with Sarah. I now felt somewhere in the middle, in a fairly balanced state. Like a pendulum that is gradually slowing down, I felt I had almost achieved a place of equilibrium. This was very comforting and I felt much stronger and more stable than before. I had not anticipated this change at all. I think I had vaguely hoped to feel better physically and less stressed through Sarah's therapy, but because I had come to her on the recommendation of someone else and hadn't really bothered to read much about her work in advance, my knowledge and expectations of what else might happen were very limited. Anyway, it's a tendency of mine to not ask too many questions and initially I had been quite sceptical. I had no idea what Sarah was doing with her gentle touch and was astonished at what that contact precipitated in me. In fact, it was very difficult to name what *had* happened. I just knew that deep inside something were very different and I was no longer feeling quite so angry or abandoned. Even identifying difficult feelings was different for me. Previously, I don't think I had enough insight to recognise what I was feeling at all. I was so used to avoiding looking at anything. All I knew was that I had been feeling ill, tired and panicky but that had now changed.

I took this new attitude home with me and once again tried it out on the family. Instead of reacting to the children's behaviour, I experimented with a slightly more laidback approach. Confusingly, their first response was to behave worse than before, but as the weeks wore on and I maintained my ground, I could see that they were finding it less and less necessary to try to wind me up, and I found that my buttons were not being pushed so frequently. The result was that I felt even more balanced.

Nigel still didn't seem to want to discuss anything to do with my physical or emotional state, so I didn't bother him with it any more and for the first time that actually felt fine. It was becoming very obvious that Nigel and I had many issues in common, which was what had attracted us in the first place, but which also had the potential to affect our relationship. However, if he was not yet ready to deal with things in his own way, my best plan would be to step back from trying to get his attention and just carry on with my own journey. My hope was that he might see how much better I was after having faced some of my own difficulties. I honestly doubted that he would follow the same path, but perhaps some alchemy might take place that would allow him to get an insight into himself in a way that was comfortable for him. I was deeply grateful to Sasha for giving me the signpost towards Sarah, and I do now believe that the bodywork approach was the best one for me. I was slowly beginning to see that it was okay to have a life of my own outside the home, where I could get to know and trust myself better instead of relying on others for self-confidence and respect. The idea of being able to hold a thought like that without getting panicky was like having a small, warm comforting space just for myself. I guess what I was experiencing was the growing ability to take care of myself without feeling that someone else was reneging on the job and that I had been dealt the short straw. My family had expected me to take care of my own emotional well-being without any input from them. Possibly because of their own experiences in childhood, they were unavailable when I needed support and attention, and so I had grown a tough but brittle outer shell, which nevertheless had a soft, needy centre. I had always felt the urge to hide and internalise my feelings because I believed that there was no one there to listen. Having Oscar as a single mother, I had to be brave and self-sufficient for him so my own needs retreated further and further down the list. I had eventually married Nigel who was caring and willing to take on Oscar, but in temperament I had chosen someone very like my mother. Like me, Nigel had difficulty with expressing or receiving emotion. I was cycling around the same problem with all the major figures in my life – parents, lover, husband – without any means of seeing or changing the pattern. My body had been taking the toll. No wonder it had been screaming for help.

That's why I arrived at my ninth session with Sarah feeling more at peace with myself. Although I still had symptoms of one sort or another, I found that I was beginning to understand more clearly the links between my early childhood experiences and the stress I had felt before. I had begun to notice how my present situation could reignite that stress and bring on symptoms like headaches or stomach cramps. In other words, I was starting to listen to my body and stop blaming it for feeling bad as if it were separate from me and completely disconnected from my feelings and actions. Now there was a union between my head and the rest of my body, and I felt much more of a whole person.

When I arrived Sarah asked how things had been going during the week. She was pleased when I told her how I was doing. She suggested that we start this session by looking at some things that I could do between appointments to help and support myself on a more permanent basis. I could see the benefit of knowing that. I would really like to be more in touch with my body and how it works, as up until now I have felt that it was pretty alien to me. I had little sense of how emotions might impact me physically and I would really like to find out how to prevent myself from falling back into unawareness.

We started with me sitting on the stool next to her mirror. Sarah put her hands lightly on my neck and once again I realised how much I was tightening and scrunching up in almost everything that I did. I wasn't aware of consciously doing this and it was only when she brought it to my attention that I saw what she meant. She kept talking as her hands moved around my neck and back, shoulders and arms. It was a new idea that I had the ability to prevent the build-up of stress and tension in my body and I had an almost staggering glimpse of freedom. Although yet again her hands didn't appear to be doing anything, I was aware of feeling completely different, somehow more solid and yet at the same time more open and free. There was no need to rush, either in my head or in my body, and I saw how much quieter everything could be. There was a deepening consciousness of the speed of my normal mental and physical reactions. Thinking about how I moved or carried myself in this sort of minute detail was surprisingly hard work and after a time we moved to the table.

Sarah told me that I should lie down once a day in the way that she would teach me. She said that by doing this regularly I would be helping to replace the habits of tightening with those of lengthening and widening. She showed me how much support my head needed so that it stayed level with my back. I had to raise my knees, which made the whole of my lower back rest more comfortably on the table. She asked me again to imagine that I was lying on a beach and to think about what kind of impression my back would make in the sand. It was a bit different to the other sessions, as I was much more a part of the process. I was surprised at how much difference you can make merely by thinking about these changes and I began to realise how difficult it was to think and not to do. The directions she gave me were quite simple and were really effective in giving me a sense of change in the body. These were things I could do at home and she said that in time they would make a difference to how I respond to my body and vice versa.

Sarah moved my limbs a lot more than she had done in previous sessions. She particularly focussed on my arms, neck and shoulders. After a while I noticed myself getting flatter and flatter on the couch; it felt as if my entire body was taking up more space and that the whole of my back seemed to be fused to the bed. When I sat up, she showed me in her mirror how straight my back had become during the session. This was an odd sensation because it felt so easy and as if I wasn't making any effort at all, yet I looked so upright.

This was definitely a different kind of session. Sarah did do some Craniosacral work towards the end, and I felt myself much more able to respond. Going out, I had a marvellous sense of being taller and freer in my body than I had ever felt before; my head was as light as a feather, floating on my neck, and my arms and shoulders seemed wider. Mentally, I felt calmer and more at ease with myself. I began to see how much unconscious strain I had been carrying over the years and hoped I would be able to maintain this sense of lightness and softness for as long as possible. Next time will be my tenth session with Sarah and I'm ready for it and what it might bring. I feel more curiosity about life in general and much less fear. This journey has helped me to start to feel brave and adventurous.

It occurred to me that this tenth session might be my last. Sarah might think I am ready to move on, and that is something to think about during the time leading up to it. I'm not sure how I feel about life without Sarah just yet; perhaps I'm not so brave and adventurous after all.

## Sarah's Story

I was pleased to see that Anna was looking far more upbeat and peaceful than she had been. There was a softness to her face and a clarity in her eyes that told me that she was more at ease with herself and life generally since our last meeting. I wanted her to continue to experience this new stability within herself and decided to give her some tools so that she could begin to develop more 'core strength'. In Craniosacral terms 'core strength' describes a strong sense of flow and organisation through the centre of the body. In an Alexander Technique lesson we are teaching the ability to direct consciously that upward flow in everyday life. We are looking to inhibit any reactions that interfere with the continuity of brain and spinal cord and which might cause disruption within the body, either locally or globally.

When Anna had arrived for her early sessions in such a distressed state I thought that initially she would benefit more from the quietness and stillness of Craniosacral work. I hoped it would give her depleted nervous system a chance to settle down before learning something new. Now she was much calmer I suggested that we start looking at ways that could help her maintain equilibrium in between our sessions. I could see from her face that I had hit a chord, since she had told me she generally felt really good and positive after the sessions but had no way of maintaining it once she had left my room. Over time it tended to dissipate slowly in the face of any stress she encountered. We can't change what we don't see, so one of my first tasks would be to encourage Anna to notice what she was doing physically. In the words of one of the early Greek Philosophers: 'How can we search for that which we do not know?' More than anything else, it was an awareness that I was hoping to encourage in her.

I started by inviting Anna to sit on a chair, feel her feet on the ground and at the same time be aware of the distance between the top of her head and the ceiling. Then I taught her how to be more conscious of her peripheral vision and the space behind her. Bit by bit I could feel her breathing change and her customary anxiety lessen. She stopped bracing her legs and holding her breath and became interested in the ongoing sensations of her body in time and space. I could feel that she was more present and able to respond to what was going on around her rather than being perpetually stuck in the revolving emotional drama in her mind. Our next step would be for Anna to be able to preserve this awareness of herself; my eventual aim was to show her how to direct her own body movement, both during our lessons and, more importantly, in her daily life. It could be described as a practical course in mindfulness. We worked in this way for a time, gradually looking at how she moved and determining whether she could allow herself to replace her usual habits with something different. I was interested to know how this would make her feel and hoped to give her the ability to choose an appropriate reaction; for instance, the muscular tension needed for picking up a paper bag is less than that needed for a heavy suitcase.

After a while I suggested that she move to the table. Here I asked her to notice and identify her emotions and their location in her body. I wanted Anna to describe those physical sensations without instantly labelling them as happy, sad, good or bad, etc. Our feelings are so intimate and familiar to us that trying to experience them afresh can be helpful. I know how quickly I can fall into well-worn paths myself. A familiar feeling tone for example nearly always produces a specific emotion, but what produces that feeling tone and does it always have to lead to that particular emotion? By asking Anna to observe herself in this way I wanted to encourage her to distance her physical self more from her emotional responses and to help her break an endless cycle.

So, what did I pick up in this session with Anna? She was much calmer overall and there was an impression of steadiness. I was able to tell that she was conscious of the length of her spine from her head down to her sacrum. I kept a similar awareness of my own spine in order to echo and amplify hers. I could still detect the familiar imprints of anxiety and fear floating around, particularly at the solar plexus, but they were not so prevalent this time. I suppose I would describe this session as a consolidation and deepening of the work that we had been doing over the previous eight sessions, and I was pleased at the way things were moving forward.

As we moved into a more Craniosacral treatment, I was thinking about how hard it is for me to define the boundaries between Craniosacral work and the Alexander Technique. As a practitioner, I suppose I could say that I move from a teaching perspective to a listening position, but this doesn't really describe the process or what someone lying on the table might feel as I move from one discipline to another. Both disciplines require me to put my hands on a pupil or client with an attitude of 'non-doing'. In the Alexander Technique we walk a fine line between trying to impart knowledge and a sensation of freedom in activity, without actually 'doing' anything. An invitation is given to move into a different relationship with yourself and your environment. As a Craniosacral practitioner I move into a more meditative space but in both therapies I try to listen and be aware not only of what is happening in my client's body but also what is happening in mine as a consequence. It's like hearing an orchestra play a piece of music. You can hear either the whole sound or the individual instruments that contribute to the sound. You can hear all at once or move from one to the other. It all depends where you place your focus and how much flexibility you allow yourself to move between layers of perception.

Towards the end of the treatment the session moved almost imperceptibly to another level that is often described by Craniosacral practitioners as the 'Long Tide'. It was an extraordinary moment for us both, and there was a profound sense of stillness in the room. Although I was fully aware of our two separate systems, I felt in that moment that Anna and I were connected at an unfathomable depth and all her areas of holding and tension seemed far off and on a completely different plane. Likes and dislikes, problems and struggles melted away and there was just the rhythm of life. It was like seeing the wider perspective from the top of a high mountain; all superficial aspects seemed to meld into each other and become part of the whole. I think Anna felt very different as she left that day, and I did too. We had connected at a level where I didn't need to rescue her or feel insecure about what I was doing, and she had enough strength to heal herself. For a moment we had become equals in our respective journeys.

## Our Story

Grant me the serenity to accept the things I cannot change, the courage to change the things I can, and the wisdom to know the difference.

*The Serenity Prayer*

### LIZ AND DAŠKA

The Serenity Prayer, used in Alcoholics Anonymous meetings across the world, implies that there is an equanimity that comes from acceptance and that if you can come to terms with the fact that you cannot change and improve everything in life, you may at least find some peace. We have found this a useful sentiment, both in our own work and lives and as advice for our clients.

Acceptance in a therapeutic context could take the following form. Someone suffering from Post-traumatic Stress Disorder can present with severe or extreme dissociation. Inviting such a client to try to experience feelings in the body without naming or judging them may be impossible because of a justifiable terror that re-inhabiting the body might bring back all the memories that they had been trying so hard to forget. In such a case, retreating from the body could not be seen as neurotic but a really successful tactic, enabling survival in what might otherwise be an impossible situation. The downside is that it could become a familiar and constant way of interacting with life and that it may no longer be possible to release overwhelming tension even when safe to do so. We have both experienced clients shaking with the effort of trying to hold things together and found that the only thing to do was to contain them in a tight embrace. It may not be possible to accept a more interpretive touch in this instance, but the practitioner might be able to encourage a sense of warmth and safety, if only temporarily. Working in this way demands acceptance by both therapist and client. For the therapist, there is the admission that you can do very little to relieve people's pain because their armouring may be the only solid thing in their lives. The client has to make the giant leap of developing trust, when all her experience tells her that trust will only lead to more pain and suffering. For some this is an impossible hurdle, and that also needs to be recognised and accepted on both sides.

Like Chiron's wound, some problems are indeed insoluble. Part of the journey towards acceptance might be to acknowledge that certain wounds really can't be healed. It is the cyclical revisiting of our old stories that allows an opportunity for them to be integrated and accepted. Sometimes, though, we have to find another way.

Like pulling a jagged shard of shrapnel from a wound, digging out a trauma and bringing it into the light can sometimes cause more damage than leaving it in place and living with it.

## DAŠKA

In my own experience of being a client and having a Craniosacral session, the following thought once came to me quite suddenly in the middle of the treatment, 'That was then, this is now and I'm still here and I've survived, not perfectly and not unscarred, but here nevertheless.' I hadn't realised what an enormous amount of energy I had been using keeping past experiences locked away. This thought was a huge step in my journey and immediately made me aware of the need to reframe my thoughts and persona. If these ancient traumas were no longer dominating my reactions, my being, then who was I? What did that feel like in my body? I felt relief as I let go of the imagined necessity of both keeping the wounds hidden and hiding from them at the same time. Turning towards instead of avoiding them meant that I could begin to accept them and they began to lose some of their authority. However, that experience was not the end. I have found that, echoing what we have been writing, some old stories have resurfaced yet again. It's true that they don't dominate as much as they used to, but they are still there and they will always be a part of me and who I am. I'm no longer trying to get rid of them; instead I'm happy to let them settle into their place as an element of the whole.

## LIZ

In my own practice I have found that from time to time I have needed to accept I may not be the most appropriate person to help a particular client. One example is a man who came to see me many years ago. He was extremely needy and we formed a strong bond over a number of sessions. I felt that I could help him and in fact we worked together for a long time. However, I gradually came to see that I had taken the place of the mother who had emotionally abandoned him very early on. The abandonment was pre-verbal, and each time my client reverted to that place we seemed to get stuck in the treatment process. I realised at last that I hadn't got the skills or ability to move him forward. I was now too invested in his recovery and had become enmeshed with him. Asking him to start psychotherapy initially felt like another abandonment but was eventually very successful. I took supervision about the situation, and it was helpful to see how my own mothering tendencies had got in the way of his progress. I wasn't the best person to help him move forward, not only because I had been unable to stop mothering him, but also because of the deep frustration I encountered when we reached that silent, stuck space. I realise now that something about it triggered an unexplored part of my own early development and meant we both came to a standstill.

It should not feel difficult to pass a client on to someone else, but it often does. It can make you feel inadequate or undertrained if you believe that you should be able to meet everyone's needs and especially so if you think that clients have been drawn to you because you have something unique to offer them. I have found, though, that clients you have to pass on, or who leave of their own accord, are often very important, perhaps because you learn so much about yourself from letting them go. As holistic practitioners we need to have a wide enough perspective to realise that we cannot be all things to all people.

Acceptance of our own strengths or limitations may mean that we have to be content at times with an uncomfortable or unexpected version of ourselves. The hotshot, cure-all therapist that we saw ourselves becoming at the beginning of our career may have to mutate into someone more humble, who is content to be doing the best she can. Conversely, a nervous, tentative practitioner who has no faith in herself can learn that her vulnerability and openness helps people more than she realises and allows her clients to express these qualities in themselves. Accepting that we can't change everybody's symptoms or lives for the better is hard but necessary. It's also sometimes difficult to believe that we have made a difference. Change often happens in the work that we do, but not everything or everyone is open to change. Where something or someone is not yet ready, we may have to either let go and forget it or just sit and wait until we see another opportunity. It's as simple as that.

Anna has reached a significant point in her ongoing treatment and is beginning to accept imperfections both in herself and Nigel. In their penultimate session Anna and Sarah have also reached a moment of equilibrium. They have covered quite a lot of ground and now have the time to assimilate their experiences. We have characterised this by describing a moment in which they drop together into a deep meditative state, which is a common feature of Craniosacral Therapy treatments. Sarah describes this beautifully and we feel it illustrates perfectly the nature of this extraordinary phenomenon.

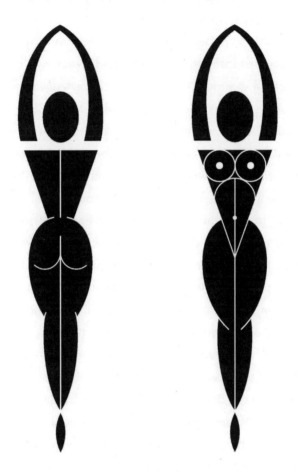

# CHAPTER TEN

# CLOSURE AND RETURN

## Anna's Story

Looking back at how I was when I first came to see Sarah, it was obvious to me that there had been meaningful changes. Many of my physical symptoms were fading and I was beginning to make better connections between those symptoms and my emotional issues. At long last I was finding a voice and an identity for myself. I no longer relied so much on others for acknowledgement and this was influencing the way I dealt with Nigel and the children, leading to some quite surprising results. Relations at home were reasonably harmonious for the first time in ages. The children seemed more settled, and Nigel and I were back on speaking terms. Although we didn't talk about my therapy with Sarah, I no longer felt I needed his approval to continue. Occasionally, I had even noticed him looking and acting more relaxed, and I hoped he was feeling better too. I think being kinder to both him and myself was making a difference. I no longer believed I was a pathetic dogsbody with a million disconnected symptoms, but instead someone who might successfully function outside the context of the family. I had even started to think about taking a part-time job while the children were at school. All of this was new, and still quite wobbly, but I was slowly beginning to believe that it was not just a flash in the pan.

My main problem now was wondering how I would manage if Sarah said she thought that our treatments were finished. I had come along with very little expectation of the therapy or of her, but over the ten sessions I had come to rely on her in many different ways. She had become very much a maternal figure, listening and responding to me unlike my actual mother. As well as that, I really liked her as a person. She seemed so wise and thoughtful, and I admired her capacity for stillness and clarity of thought. I would really miss her and I had begun to worry about how I would deal with the separation. I had gone through separations before, and they had been searingly painful. My parents' divorce and Steve's abandonment when I was pregnant had been so traumatic that I didn't want to go through that again. I felt sure that Sarah wouldn't just cut me off – I trusted her enough for that – but I wondered what she might suggest for the future. I didn't know how things worked in this kind of situation; maybe she had other clients who needed her attention now. I wondered whether they were all going through similar journeys and I noticed that I was almost becoming envious of them. It hadn't entered my head until recently that there were other people who went to see her. Of course I knew it intellectually; last time I had almost bumped into someone who was just leaving as I was arriving, and that had really brought home to me that I wasn't Sarah's only client. There was an underlying uneasiness to that knowledge since I was anticipating an end to our sessions. I was surprised at the strength of my reactions.

When I got to Sarah's, she began by summing up from her perspective how she thought things had gone over our last nine sessions. She was happy that I had made such good progress and said that she thought this might be a good moment to take a break for a short while. However, she pointed out that it was important this should also be my decision, and I should choose how I wanted to proceed. I was surprised because I had not even considered that it might be up to me. As far as I was concerned, Sarah was the expert, and I had expected her to decide how we would go forward. I suppose this was another example of always expecting that others would make decisions for me. Paradoxically, in the past, this had always left me feeling hurt and resentful. I thought for a moment and realised that if I had a choice, I would like to continue seeing Sarah regularly, but perhaps not as frequently as before. This would give an opportunity to continue exploring with the therapy and leave the space between sessions to process things for myself.

This felt like a grown-up decision, more so because I had made it on my own. Sarah agreed that this was a good way forward. Since it was now close to Christmas, we decided that there would be a natural break in any case and we would leave it for about a month or so before continuing.

The session began as usual. Settling into treatment has become much easier as the weeks have gone by. I am more and more able to sink down and relax on the table in a way that would have been unimaginable before and I have become used to bringing my attention to my body. I noticed that my shoulders were hunching up a bit, but I was able to let the shoulder blades sink down my back and move apart. This freedom made me realise that I no longer felt so vulnerable and exposed. The rest of my back softened too and I gradually felt myself moulding comfortably into the couch; my breath became longer and slower. I felt as if I could go off to sleep.

However, I didn't go to sleep, or at least not consciously. I just lay there feeling relaxed and safe. Safety is a new and interesting sensation. If you had asked me a couple of months ago what it felt like, I'm not sure if I would have been able to answer. I don't think I would even have been aware that I had no experience of safety. I believe I had long been deeply unconscious of what I needed or how I felt about things. The trauma I had suffered had produced a disconnected condition, rendering me out of touch with my own feelings. I was frozen into passive acceptance, believing that this was what life was like. Nothing in my early childhood had given me a sense of security; everything seemed to be fraught with danger. Things could change at the drop of a hat; all was random and there was never an explanation. I believed I must keep quiet so that no emotion should escape to annoy or upset other people. You have to feel safe to be able to express emotion. At a very early age I had become self-sufficient and in charge of my own emotional well-being. Nobody in my family had any idea how to provide protection either for themselves or me. My childhood experience had left me without a meaningful sense of being looked after, and the world had looked frightening and dark. Now I had a growing new perspective. Excitingly, I appeared to be gradually emerging from the deep tunnel that had shaped and restricted me for so long. Finding safety within felt warm and empowering; I was enjoying it.

The rest of the session went by quickly, and before I knew it, Sarah was announcing that it was almost time to finish. I was really sorry that I wouldn't be seeing her for a few weeks, but because I knew that there was an ongoing relationship, I didn't feel abandoned. The fact that I had made my own decision about how often I wanted to see her had given me more control than I had ever had before. I could feel a growing confidence about being able to make more decisions in the future. Finally I was growing into an adult. The frightened little girl who had grown up too fast without a support system was no longer the dominant force. I was emerging as a more grounded individual who was finding new inner strength for tackling life's problems.

Sarah had helped me to do this, and I will always be grateful to her for that. Looking back on our sessions together, I remember how confused and angry I had sometimes been that I wasn't getting any better. Sarah was wise enough to see my healing potential but knew that it could take a long time. I had blanked out those raw and painful deep memories and I had now begun revisiting them in order to lay them to rest. I had a much better sense of where I needed to go and how to get there. I am so glad now that Sarah helped me to decide to stick with the therapy over a period of time, because without her support there might have been a danger of retreating back to my disassociated self. I am now feeling much stronger although I am aware that there will be bumps in the road ahead, moments when my fragility will return. I have seen that the same lessons need to be learned over and over again and that I will still need someone to turn to when the going gets tough. I realise too how much further there is to go in this quest for wholeness we are following together, but I feel this is a moment to rest and sit at the top of this small hill before I begin to tackle the rest of the journey. I left Sarah's room looking ahead to Christmas with the family and to resuming my work with her in the New Year with a sense of optimism and hope.

## Sarah's Story

We had now come to the tenth session. Anna came into the room smiling but looking a bit distracted. I was interested to hear how she felt the treatments had gone and how she wanted to proceed. Part of our work was to help her to stand on her own two feet and I thought that it would be useful for her to take a break before continuing. As it was Christmas there would be a natural pause in any case, but I knew that it was important for Anna to make a conscious choice for herself. She seemed bemused by my asking what she wanted to do, and I could see that she hadn't yet considered that it would be up to her to choose and was expecting me to tell her what to do. In the end we agreed to speak in the New Year to arrange the next session and to continue in the future on a less intensive basis.

Anna's body had a different feel, a different texture. No wonder she had felt so uncomfortable in the past; there had been so many conflicting tensions in her body pulling her in opposing directions. Rather than an overriding impression of defeat and collapse there was instead a buoyancy and a lightness; a willingness to explore and an enthusiasm for life that had been buried before. One of the features of depression or stress is to be stuck in a cycle where you feel helpless and powerless. When we start to be more conscious of what we are doing and whether we are responding appropriately and usefully to events, we can see more clearly if we are revolving round the same old loop. What had struck me most during the sessions with Anna was the extraordinary moment when she was able to turn her story around completely. Offering her mother support rather than asking for it for herself was totally unexpected. I have thought about that a lot since and continue to be surprised and humbled by that reaction. I think I have learnt a lot from my clients over the years, but it has never been quite so dramatic or so clear.

My impression today was of a sensation of flow from the top to the bottom of her spine. It seemed as good a place as any for us to break for the moment. I was interested to see how she would cope with the stresses and strains of a family Christmas without the prop of the weekly therapy session. I hoped that I had given her enough simple techniques to be able to take a step back and look after herself when things got too demanding and overwhelming, but I did recognise that this was a tough call with a young family. I suggested that she could call me if she felt that things were getting on top of her and that we would start again in the New Year.

Throughout the session Anna seemed stronger and calmer, both physically and emotionally. She had obviously been able to come to a better place in her relationships with both Nigel and her children, and this showed in her body. We had a very simple treatment, and Anna seemed oddly both very present and one step removed. I think she may have been getting used to the fact that we won't be seeing each other for a few weeks and was unconsciously separating herself slightly. Her adult self is guiding her well now that her 'inner child' feels more supported and secure. I shall miss the small Anna who needed my help to get this far, but I look forward to working with a more grown-up woman in the New Year.

Later that evening I reflected over the course of the work with Anna. She will never know how much I have learned and gained from our encounter; at times it really did feel like a 'joint practice'. I wish I could share this with her, but of course I can't and I won't. I have begun to have much more confidence in my work and in being able to trust my instincts; I know that this is something that Carol has been trying to encourage for years, but words alone are not enough. Anna's vulnerability and the fact that her story touched me so deeply, combined with the unexpected reappearance of my own family saga, all united over a few sessions to produce a healing of sorts for both of us. I had been in such an emotional turmoil myself that I had had no choice but to let go of everything and just trust that my gut feeling was sound and would carry us through. It did and created a body of work that fed us both.

I have begun to rediscover the magic that first attracted me to this work; the extraordinary mixture of complete groundedness and embodiment combined with the numinous that I have found in no other field. The odd thing was that I discovered this by contravening all the training I had done – I know that I have a tendency to mother my clients and that this can lead to 'smothering' and not allowing them to take responsibility for themselves, but in this instance it was exactly what Anna had needed for her to move forward. I know too that this hasn't altered the fact that I will always need to be aware of the inclination to take on too much both in my work and in my life. I saw the truth of what Carol has been trying to teach me – that each moment requires something different – and it was only by being open to it rather than arriving with sets of preconceptions about how to work that something mysterious could enter. I have to say that unless I had been forced into that place by external circumstances, I would probably not have got there on my own, but I did and I will take that knowledge with me. Anna's moment of insight continues to affect me. She has become part of my story as I will be part of hers.

## Our Story

### LIZ AND DAŠKA

Sarah and Anna have agreed to cut back their sessions after Christmas, because it feels like a good time to bring the more intensive part of their journey to a close. Endings are always difficult, whether in the therapeutic context or in general life. They have to be negotiated carefully to avoid feelings of shock, bereavement or abandonment. Sarah and Anna have had an intense and meaningful relationship over a period of time but are now reaching a place of transition. The weekly sessions are coming to an end, and a new routine will be replacing them. The break of about a month over Christmas is the longest time Anna has gone without an appointment with Sarah since the start of the sessions. Although their therapeutic relationship is not coming completely to an end, it is changing, and Anna will be testing her wings over the holidays, often a time when stress levels are raised and challenged anyway. It's possible that over this period Anna might feel a little like a bird ejected too early from the nest, but Sarah has given her the opportunity of checking in if necessary.

Sarah might also find some difficulties with this new situation. Over the course of their work she has been intimately witnessing Anna's life and experiences. Her self-acknowledged need to rescue has come out of the closet more than once. She will probably find herself thinking and worrying about Anna's ability to cope without the regular sessions. Endings can be as hard for the practitioner as for the client, particularly a client one has come to like or admire. It is easy to feel that you would like your client to keep coming for longer than they need to. It's never clear-cut and sometimes motives can be muddled.

If we look at Anna and Sarah's story through the window of mythology again, we can see how much it parallels the story of Demeter and Persephone. We could view the tale as being one related to the change and transition from carefree youth to the responsibilities and concerns of maturity. In life as in the myth, this can be a violent awakening, particularly as our culture has lost the rituals that were once used to signify these passages or transitions. It is not that these transitions no longer exist; it is that we have lost the symbolic ways of honouring and preparing for them. Although she has children of her own, Anna has tended to react from a childlike place; she has not been able to shake off her early experiences or shed the perspectives of youth. Anna has now started to tackle the buried remnants of the past, which were still colouring her approach to life. Untreated, her symptoms might well have led to a breakdown. Anna had been desperately looking to Nigel for the support so lacking in her childhood but this wasn't in his power to give. It was time for her to put away childish things and to assume a new role within her family and within society as a whole. Sarah holds that intention and offers Anna the space and time to choose a different direction.

Like Anna, Persephone needed to go into the deep, dark, hidden places in her psyche before she could emerge with a recognition of her own needs and the ability to give them a voice. The myth is an ancient way of describing the process of mental breakdown and subsequent regeneration. What we have always liked about this way of perceiving breakdown is the fact that no blame or shame is ascribed to the one who breaks down. To the contrary, it is either a significant rite of passage, as it has been for Anna, or a process foisted upon us by something entirely beyond our comprehension.

In the mythological world, protagonists are frequently subject to indiscriminate forces completely outside their control. They might find themselves at the whim of some random god or goddess and it is only when those gods are appeased that they can be released from their suffering.

Demeter is distraught at the loss of her daughter to the darkness of Hades and brings all her skills to bear in the rescue of Persephone. In time, Persephone returns to the upper world a wiser woman, but one who recognises that she will need to return to her own depths from time to time. However, she is now revered as queen of the underworld, and this gives her a new-found confidence and poise.

For those who have experienced physical or emotional trauma, the body itself may play the role of Hades, the dark and mysterious place where the unspeakable is lodged and which we fear to enter. We may be unaware that our physical self can also be a source of wisdom or support. Once we begin to explore the wisdom of our body and its felt sense in a safe and supported environment, we may discover its inherent potential for healing our wounds. We find that we may have a new perspective on pain and how to deal with it. When Anna first came to see Sarah, her body was a mysterious and scary place. Through Sarah's gentle touch and in a secure space she began to explore the darkness of early memories that had been calcified in her tissues for many years. As her body began to give up its stories, she recognised them as her own and saw the power that they had long held over her whilst they remained concealed. With growing confidence she was beginning to accept her body and see herself in a more adult light without the fear and disconnection she had always experienced.

A therapist such as Sarah would probably want to review the whole experience with her supervisor, to discuss how she worked, what she was trying to do, where she might have been helpful and how she might have worked differently. In reality, the journey that we show Anna undertaking is relatively rare, but it does happen and it is encounters like these that make our work so rewarding. Sarah discovered that, like Perceval in the myth, trusting her intuition was the key to facilitating the work with Anna. Perceval has to put aside his early patterning that taught him never to ask questions. He was able at last to stand on his own two feet and allow his spontaneous compassion to rise to the surface.

Sometimes a client may be looking for support from someone whom she perceives as stronger and more knowledgeable than she is herself. In the early stages until they can meet on common ground, a therapist may have to play a parental role to gain a client's trust. Being too invested in the part, however, can mean that the client doesn't get the chance to emerge as an adult. In our fiction, Sarah subtly draws back over time, and Anna is now more equipped to mother herself.

So, what is the long-term goal of this therapeutic encounter and what are the peaks and troughs of therapy? In some ways we are aiming for our clients to move from fixity and rigidity to adaptation and fluidity, and this is, we hope, what we show. Our protagonists are respectively quite pleased with where they have got to, but Anna's present stability is relatively fragile and will need more reinforcement to bring about lasting change. Physical habits can reflect and perpetuate our emotional and mental outlook. Change has to occur on many levels at once or old physical habits will simply creep back in, dragging with them their emotional counterparts or vice versa. Anna is growing up; she is discovering that life isn't fair. She is confronting her belief systems. This work is never finite; her questioning and conclusions will need to be revised in the future if she is to continue to develop. Answers and belief systems that suit a teenager are very unlikely to satisfy a middle-aged woman who, through the challenges she has encountered along the way, has lost some of the illusions of her youth. Disillusionment starts with separation from the mother, progresses through discovering that Father Christmas isn't real and so it goes on.

It is a hard fact of therapy that many issues are never completely resolved but recur throughout our lives in different forms and circumstances. It is hoped that what therapy gives us is the skill to negotiate our problems in a new way. It gives us another angle. We are better resourced through the work to withstand the traumas we may have suffered with more stamina and understanding. If we have a weak digestive system for example, it will probably remain something that we need to be conscious of throughout life. We will need to know what foods to eat, how much and how often in order for us to function efficiently. Similarly, in our psychological and emotional lives, we might always be susceptible to thinking, feeling or behaving in particular ways. Perhaps certain triggers may always be dangerous for us. Although we might learn to recognise them and take evasive action before they become embedded they can never be entirely eradicated. It is our task to learn how to deal with these tripwires and this can only become easier when we are better equipped to do so.

People don't always heal in the way that we show with Anna. In our story we show her going through a process of bringing the unconscious into consciousness. Sometimes clients have no connection to painful memories but their physical symptoms nonetheless improve. Occasionally, someone will remember an old forgotten injury, which disappears spontaneously as you treat her, but there doesn't appear to be any connection to an accompanying emotion. One of us had a client who had been an athlete. During the treatment and as the work moved around his body, he revisited a number of old injuries that he had long forgotten; there wasn't any associated emotional component, just a recognition and an acknowledgement of the events.

To conclude, Anna has found some inner strength through her sessions with Sarah. Her body has let go of much of the tension it was holding at the beginning and her mental health has benefitted. She has found that her symptoms have improved. She has a fast-developing new attitude towards her family and to the experiences she has suffered during her life. The fog is lifting. Sarah has also learned some lessons about the way she conducts her practice. She has looked into her own vulnerability and seen that she needs her clients as much as they need her. But she has also seen the importance of maintaining strong boundaries and yet being able to hold them lightly. Although she knew this before intellectually, she has been given another opportunity to truly embody it.

And what have we, individually, gained from bringing these two women to life and writing their story that will help us on our own paths? We have been midwives to this tale bringing it into the light and, as this story ends, we find ourselves like mothers whose children have flown the nest but who now find themselves more comfortable as the heroines of their own stories. We have both noticed an unexpected increase in self-confidence in our creativity and a greater awareness and acceptance of our respective strengths and weaknesses.

## LIZ

Every word of both Anna and Sarah's stories has resonated with me in my own life and practice. I have experienced the ups and downs that Sarah has in her work and the pain that Anna has felt in her body. What I was writing was familiar but, at the same time, useful to revisit. I believe that every bodyworker, whether brand new or with years of experience, can learn something from Anna and Sarah. I have learnt a great deal more about standing back and letting things emerge. As the book took shape, it seemed to be writing itself. Often I would describe something, only for a client to tell me that exact same story very soon afterwards. It was almost as if I was being directed to describe a particular scenario only to see it confirmed in real life. There seemed to be a magic afoot that replicated the synchronicity of the work itself.

What has been amazing and heartening to me is how we have been able to edit each other's work freely without conflict. We were each able to see how a sentence could be phrased better or a paragraph moved without suffering bruised egos. As in our Craniosacral work we have seen that the greater good is more important than an individual agenda.

Whilst writing this book we have played out all three of the female parts in the Demeter myth. We set out on the journey without any idea of how to put it all together. Like Persephone we innocently gathered thoughts to make a random bunch of ideas, trusting that somehow things would work out. As time went on, we also lived the Demeter role. We went searching for our book, sometimes in dark places, so that we could bring it into the daylight. Like Demeter's retreat from life, I too withdrew from the world during the writing process; my own practice was much quieter than usual and friends noticed I was less communicative.

Finally, we found Hecate, or the crone part of ourselves. Hecate is often depicted as a witch, but her contribution to our book is that of bringing the maturity and wisdom of years as well as the element of magic to the story. As a goddess she is associated with crossroads and transitional places, and she accompanied Persephone on her return to Hades acting as her companion and guide. She is the light-bearer who illuminates the dark place with her twin torches, and we have found that her presence has informed our task of throwing light on the magical elements of the work we do. It has been interesting to watch different aspects of ourselves emerging and to recognise that they have all been there from the beginning, just waiting for their moment to come on stage.

Working closely with another person to produce something with which you are both happy could easily have been a challenge. Instead it was an opportunity for me to look in depth at my ability to either lead or follow and to experience the subtleties of collaboration. Again this runs parallel to my work as a Craniosacral Therapist and has been invaluable as well as truly enjoyable.

## DAŠKA

Like Liz, I too have found the writing of this book has been a parallel process to those of both Anna and Sarah. It has meandered around and in reviewing the text I am often unsure who originally wrote which piece. My own life and practice has in some shape or form echoed what we have been writing – not always exactly, but at times it has almost been identical. I have often wished that I could listen to my own words; it all seems so wise on the page and yet, as we hear Sarah say in Chapter Six, my life feels a good deal messier than the one we represent in our fiction. I suppose that this was one of the areas we originally set out to explore. No one, at least in any of the books that I had read, managed to explain what it really felt like to be a therapist. How does it feel when you are not sure of either the work itself or your abilities as a practitioner? What happens if you are working with a person whose story is not only close to your own, but whose issues you also share but haven't resolved for yourself? Writing this has helped me look again at all those assumptions that I thought were universal only to discover that they turned out to be mine alone.

We also wanted to give a flavour of the potential of this magical, mysterious and wonderful work. I think that this has been the greatest challenge, as bodywork is by its nature conveyed through sensory experience, and it does not make sense to the logical and overpowering mind. Like Nigel, I have struggled with this aspect in the past. How can someone just putting her hands on someone make any conceivable difference either to her mental state or to any physical symptoms that she may have? In essence I think I was asking, how can this work be effective when I can't understand it? And yet, it is and has changed the course of my life and for that I will be eternally grateful. Like both Anna and Sarah, I think that one of my main learning curves has been an acceptance of the fact that *I don't know*, either as a therapist or as a client.

Bodywork is not a universal panacea. It is not appropriate for everyone or every condition. It is just one avenue open to exploration, but one that can have far-reaching consequences and can open up completely unexpected ways of seeing and interacting with the world.

### LIZ AND DAŠKA

We have a great fondness for myths of all cultures. However much we read them they continue to resonate and 'live' in new ways. Instead of being external tales that have no real connection to our 21st-century existence, they are to be found in all of our bodies. They are roadmaps showing ways in which each of us might face the challenges of our lives. Joseph Campbell, as ever, puts it more succinctly:

> The latest incarnation of Oedipus, the continued romance of Beauty and the Beast, stand this afternoon on the corner of Forty-second Street and Fifth Avenue waiting for the traffic lights to change.

In the classic myth of Theseus and Ariadne, the hero Theseus finds himself abandoned within the labyrinth facing the Minotaur. Because of its obvious symbolism this myth has been used many times as a metaphor for the internal journey. Theseus has to descend to the underworld to face the monster who is half man and half beast. We too may have to descend into our underworlds, our unconscious, in order to assimilate the unknown within us, our shadows, and the hidden parts of us that are not rational. Like Theseus, we can only tame or disarm the monster by confronting it. In the myth, the Minotaur is fed by a steady supply of innocent young men and women, just as we continue to feed the monster if we keep ignoring instead of facing it.

The underworld is a labyrinth; if Theseus succeeds in killing the Minotaur there is no guarantee that he will be able to find his way out. He cannot reason his way out; there is no logic here that will provide him with clues to escape. We cannot power our way through our unconscious, our shadow sides, using intellect only. The myth shows us that the masculine is only half of the story; we must accept and integrate the feminine and learn that logic and reason are not the only tools available to us. Theseus is not led out of the labyrinth; he is given the means to find his own way out by Ariadne, but must do the work himself. She gives him a thread that he can fasten to the entrance of the labyrinth, which allows him to retrace his steps, so finding his way back from the underworld.

After the escape from the labyrinth, Theseus and Ariadne elope but she is soon abandoned on the nearby island of Naxos while Theseus sails on to further adventures alone. His is the archetypal masculine, heroic path.

On the face of it this could be read as a tale of male treachery and deceit. But on another level, of course, we do need to leave those who save us in order to pursue our own journeys.